Sunflower Kid

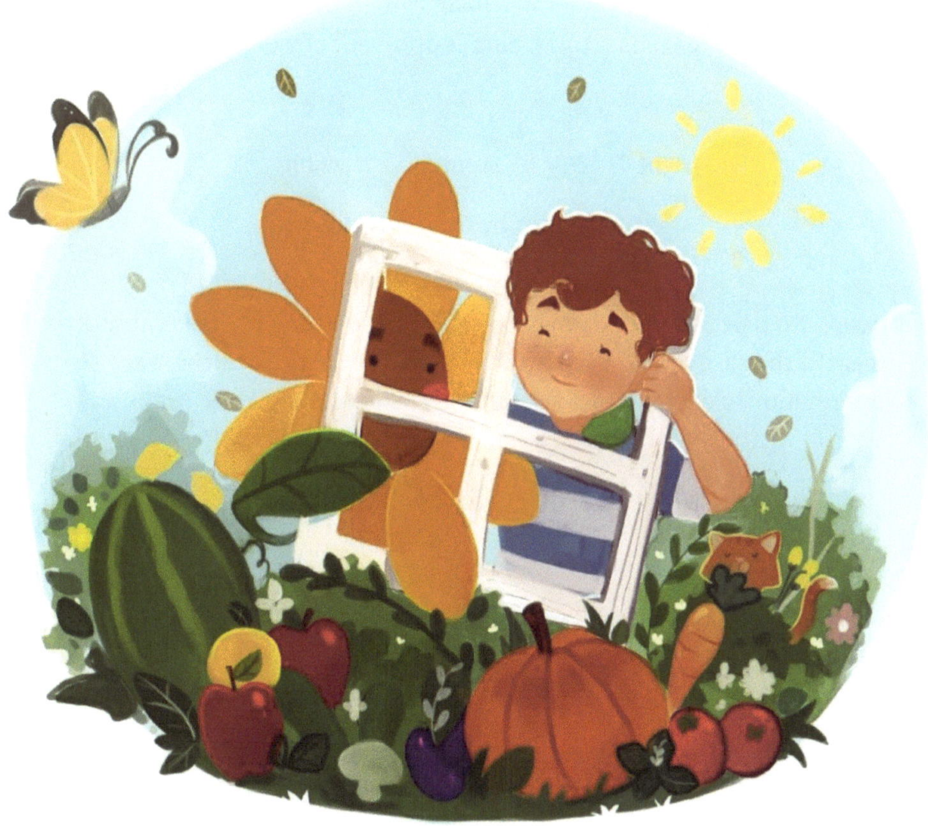

By
Stephen Bedwell Jr.

DEDICATION

To the sunflowers

Who make us stop, smile and sit in wonder

"Wake up! Wake up sleepy head!"
Mom tries to wake me out of bed.
"Remember, who will you see?"
Oh yeah! It's a weekend with Uncle and Auntie.

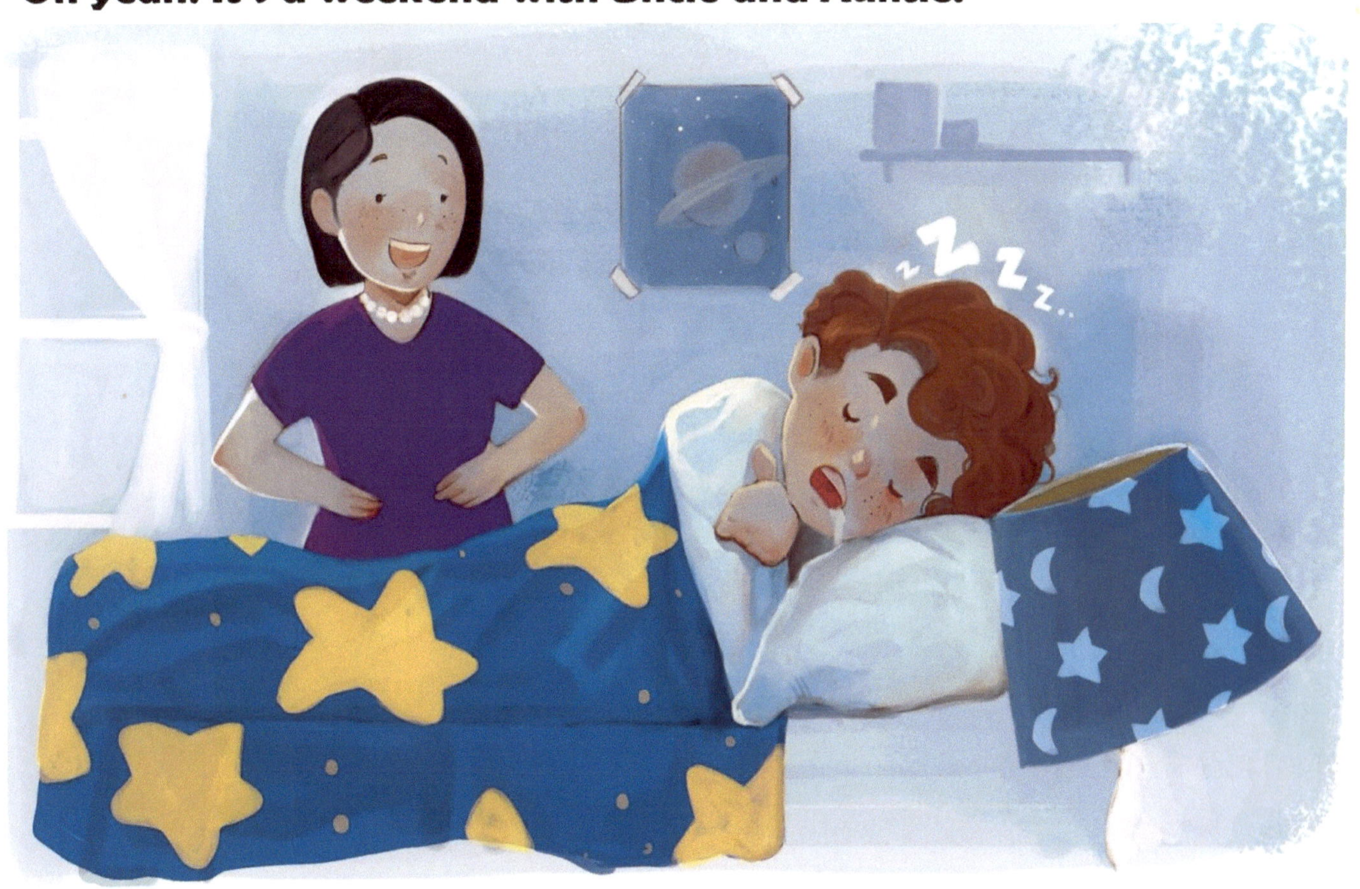

Traveling, traveling, here we go.
What will I see? I just don't know?

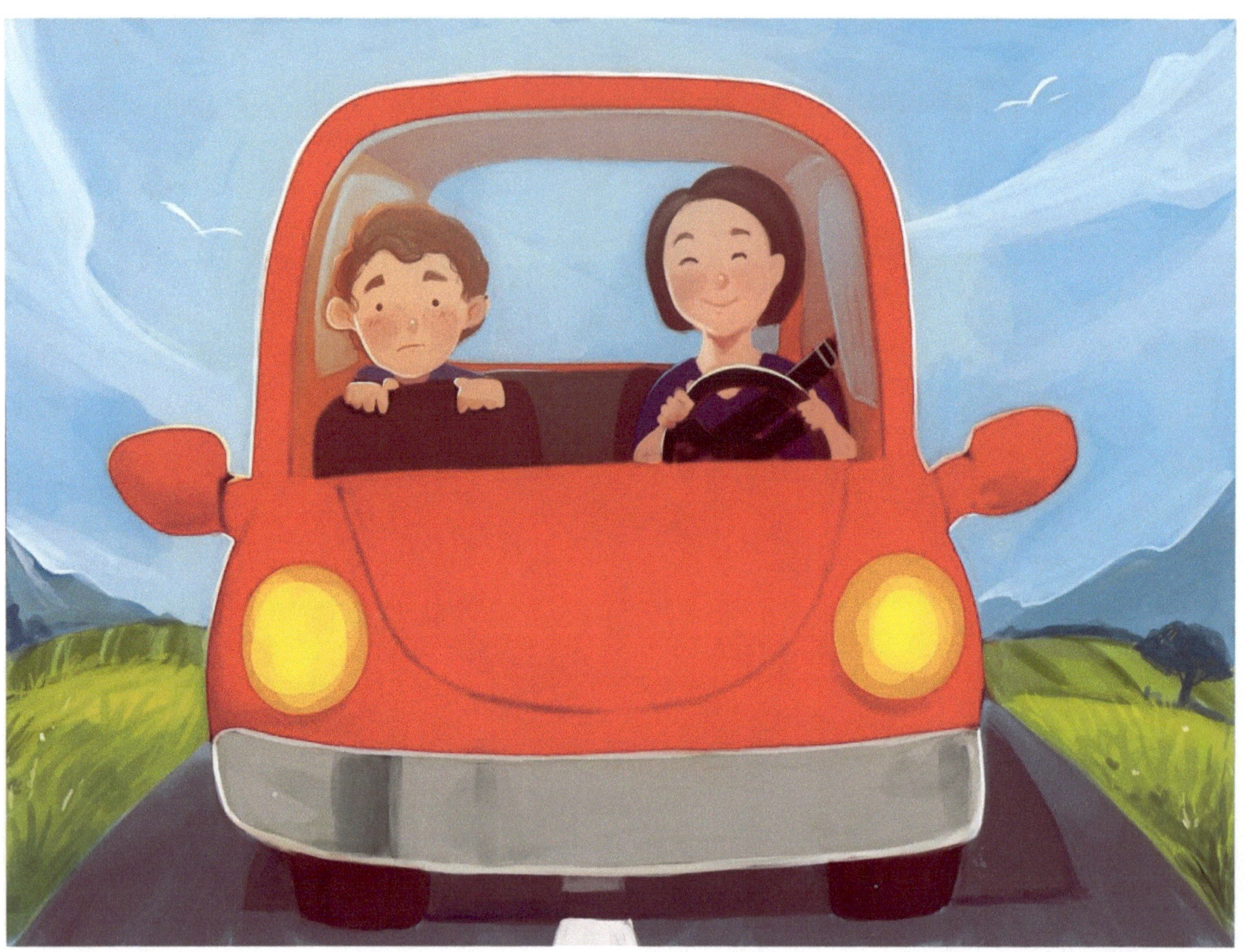

Mom says they're different than she and me.
I can't wait to see my uncle and auntie.

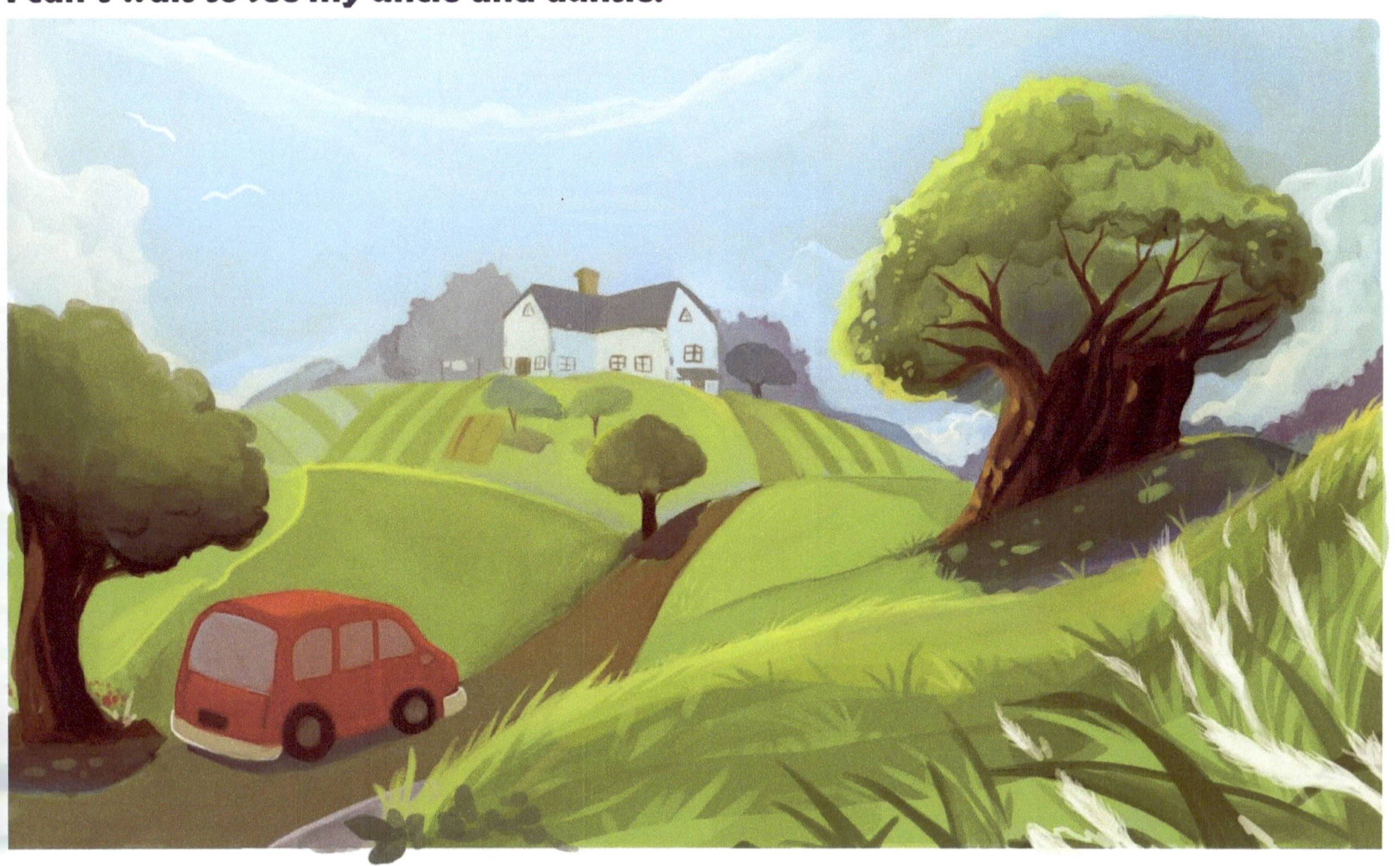

I hide like an owl amongst the leaves and branches of a tree.
And dodge around behind mom's knee.
My eyes. My eyes. They are so wide.
I just might be in for a wild ride.

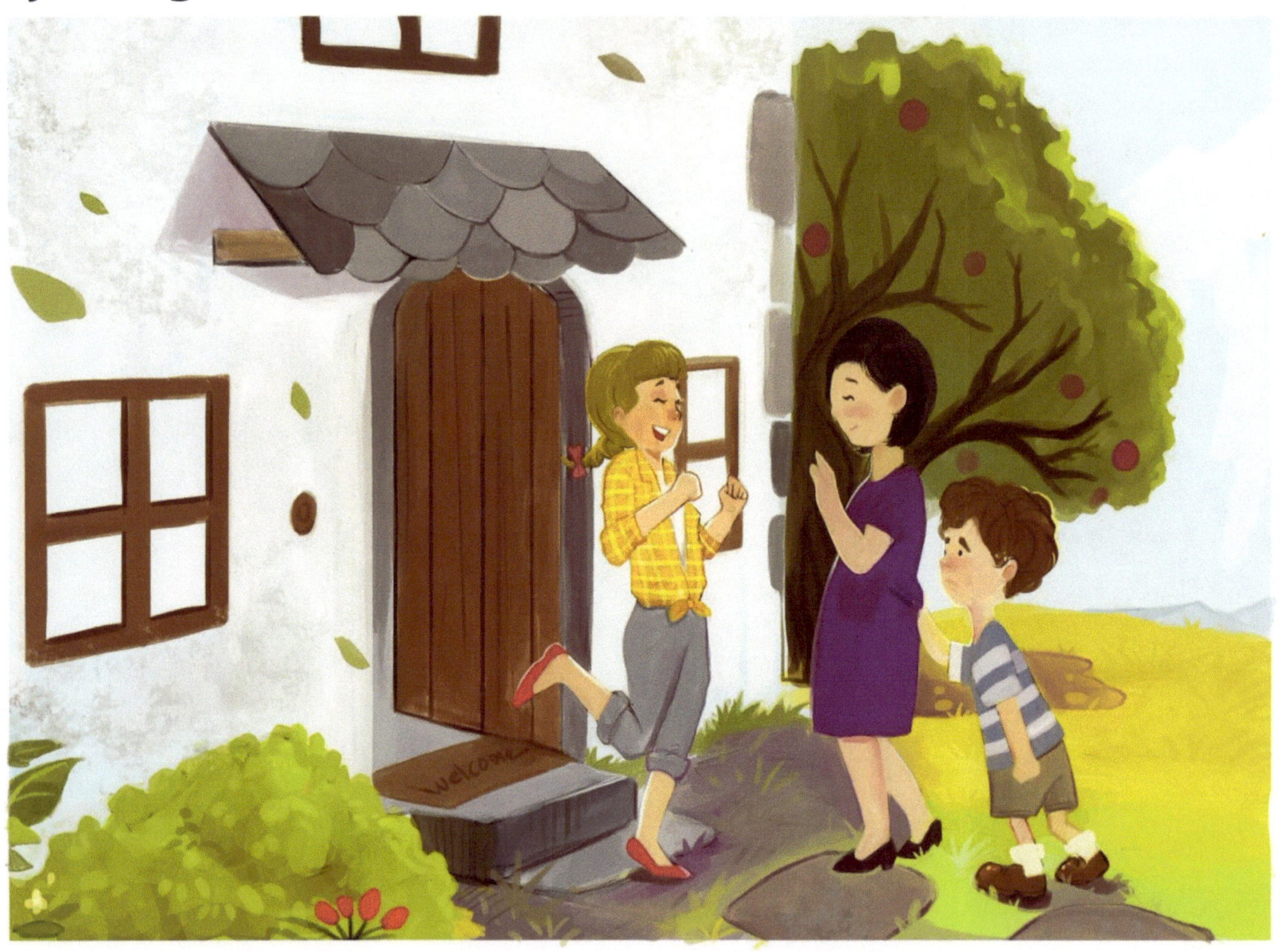

A Yurt! A Yurt! This house is a yurt.
No harm to the Earth to make it.
It nicely rests in the dirt.

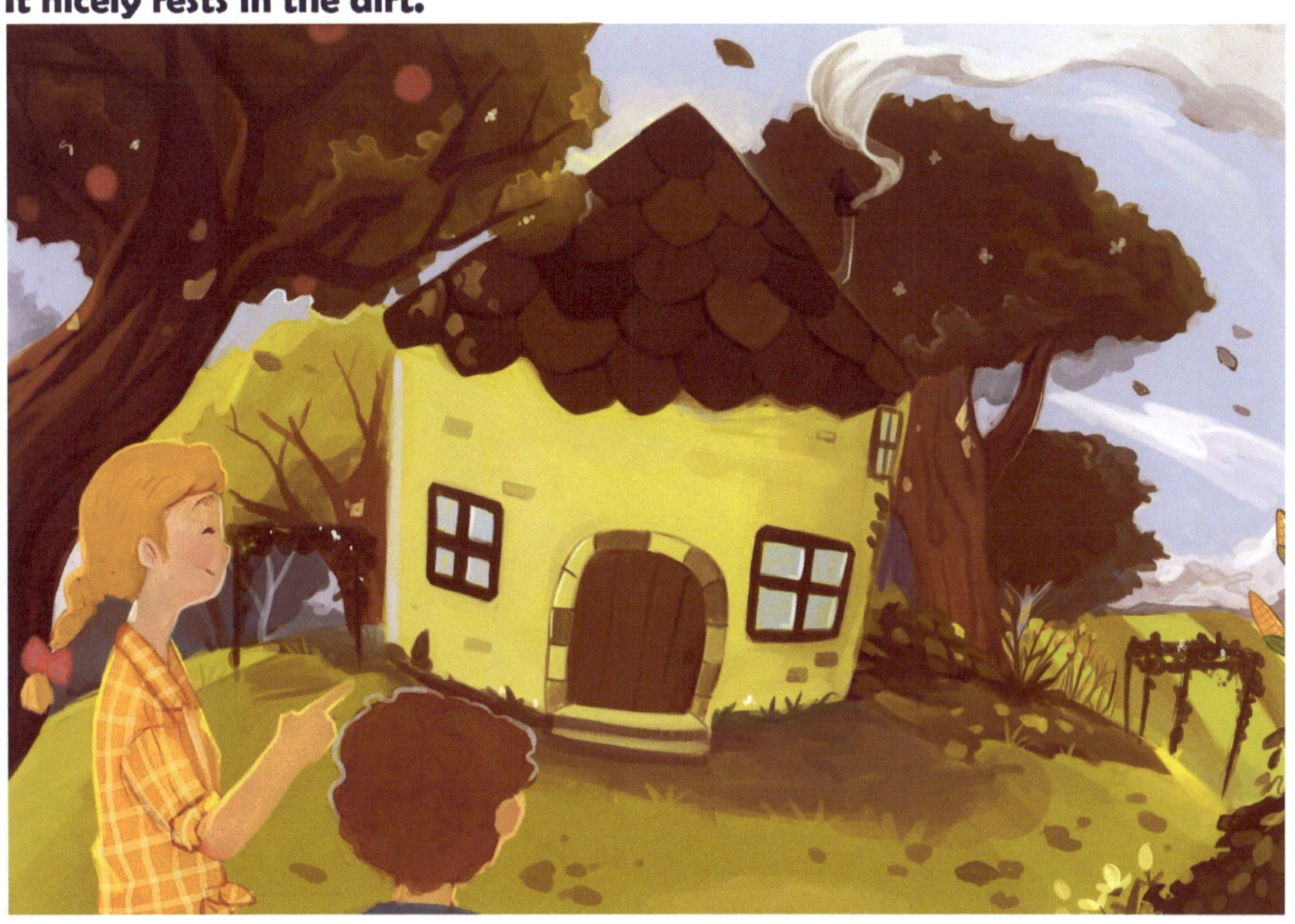

I'm a bit hungry after the long ride.
Auntie says, "Look at what I just picked from outside."

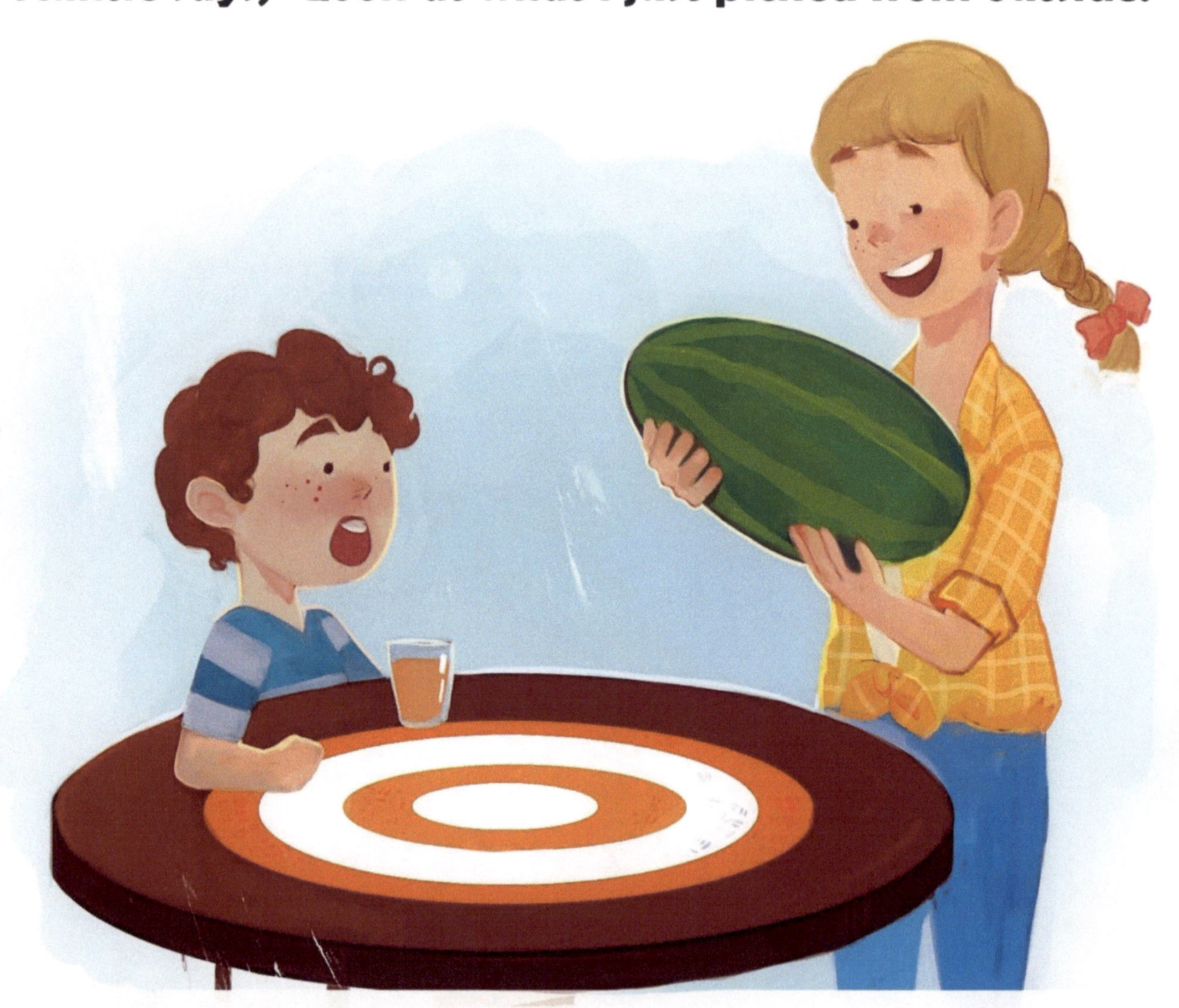

Herbs and vegetables are planted in the ground.
Uncle sneaks up on me without making a sound.
He has been outside working hard.
Just look at all the planting done in the yard.

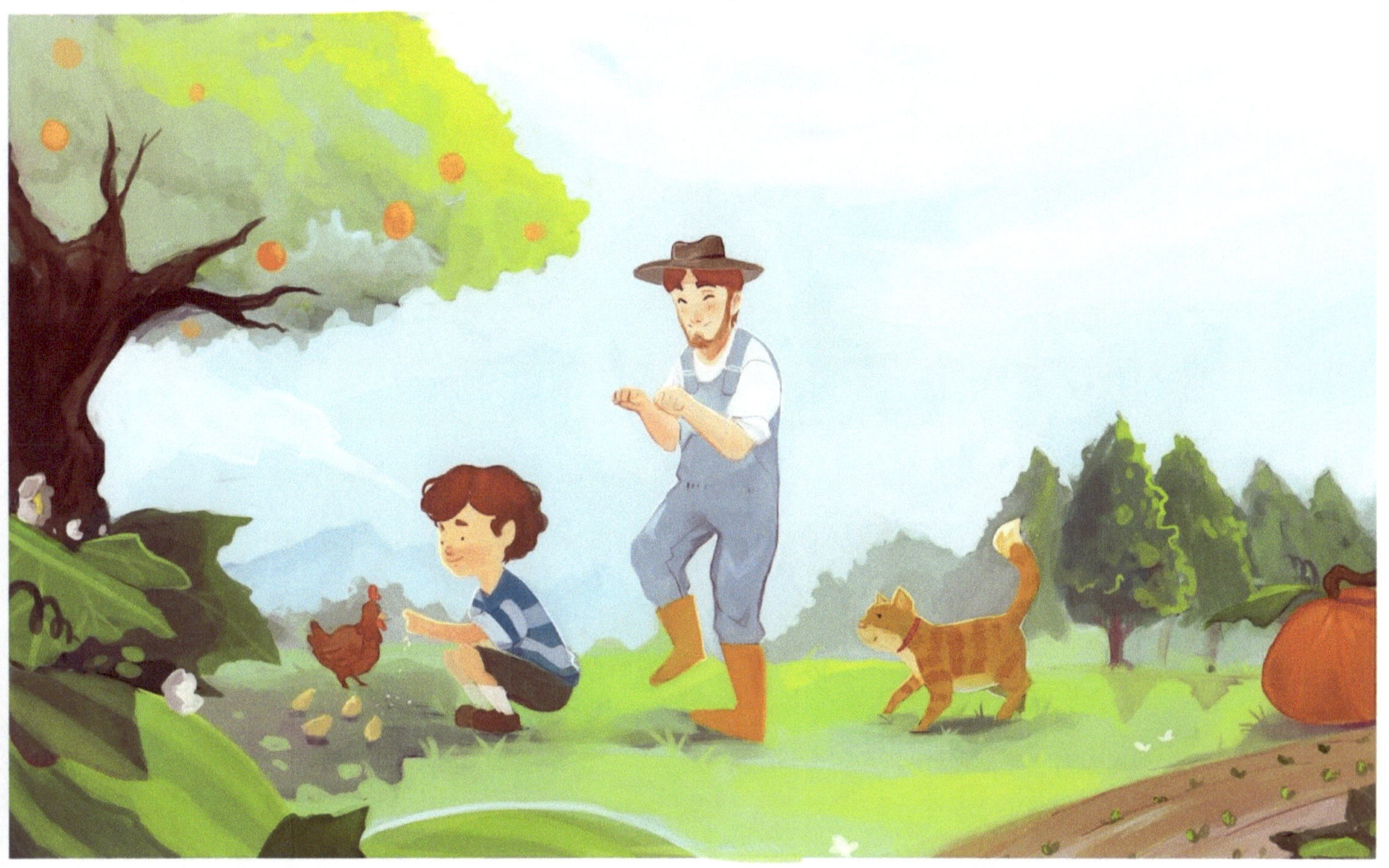

Watermelon! Watermelon! How thirst quenching you are!
Far better than anything that would come in a jar.
I can cut it in half and eat it with a spoon.
Doesn't matter if it takes me until noon.
Look at uncle with his hands covered in dirt.
He has gotten watermelon all over his face and shirt!

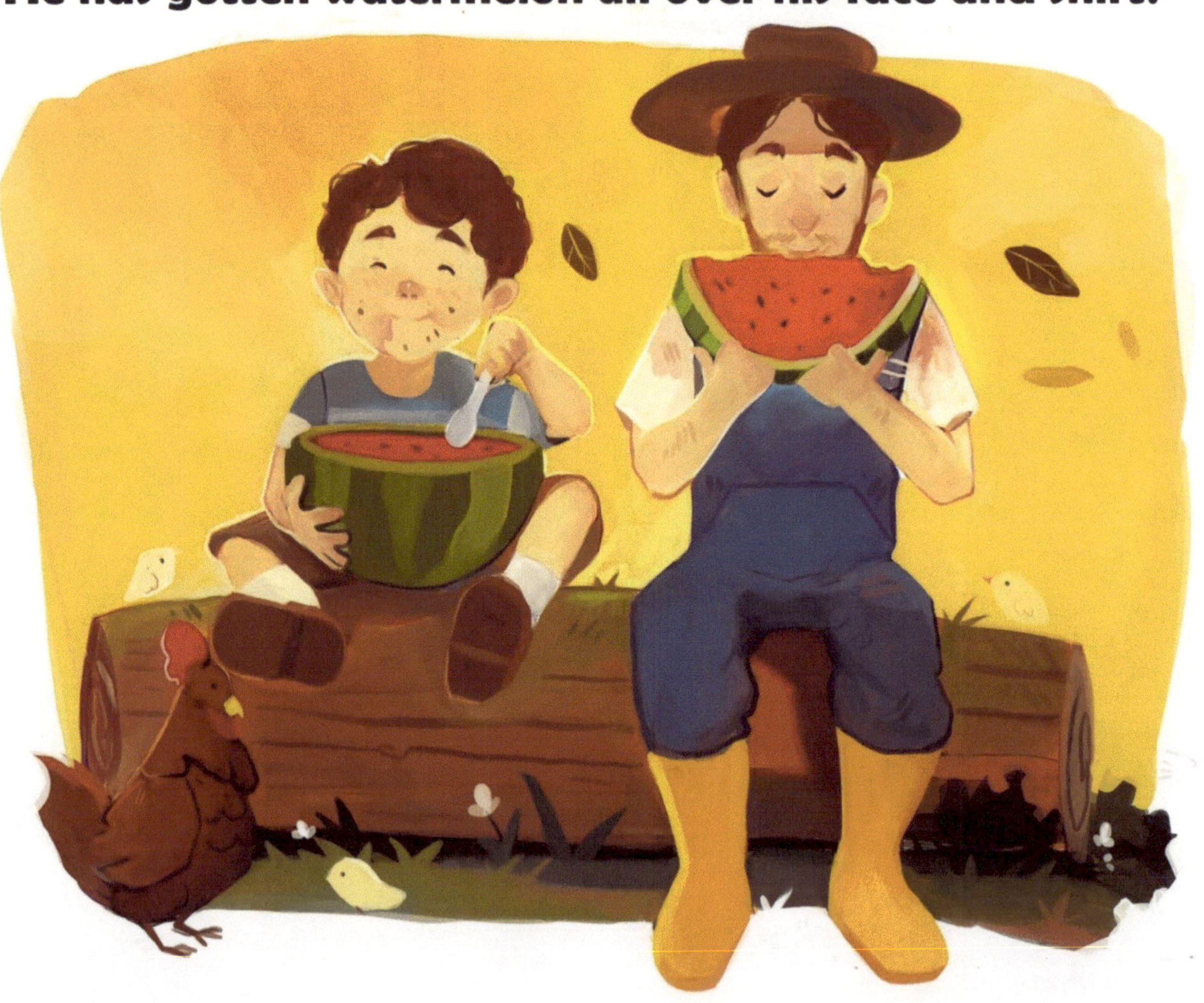

Here it is! My room for the night.
A bed to be tucked into nice and tight.
Fun echoes from the fan.
Auntie asks, "Do you know how that is ran?"

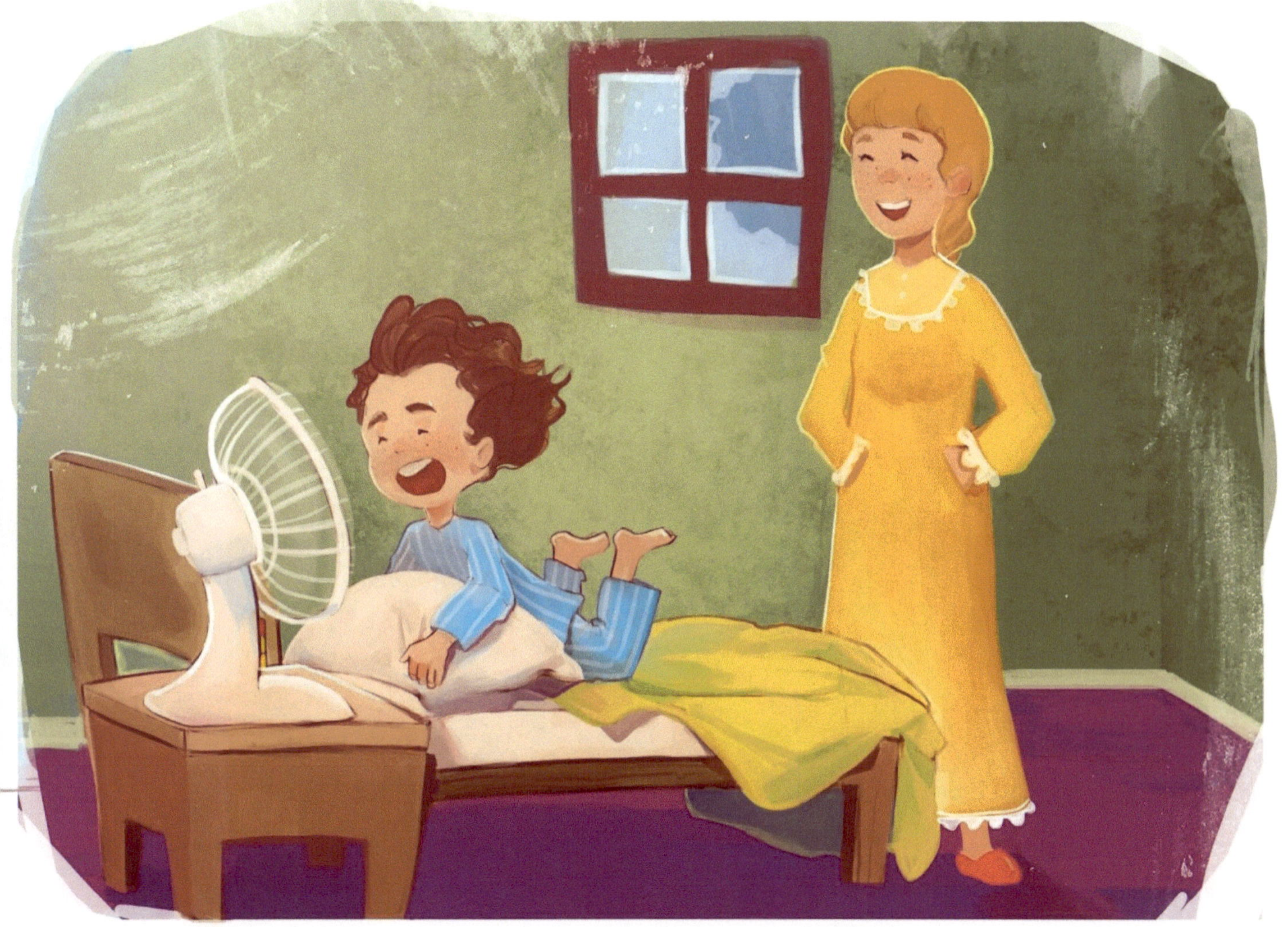

Up on the roof, solar panels lie.
Collecting sunlight, they provide energy. That is why!
Solar panels give lots of power.
You can wash your socks and take a shower.

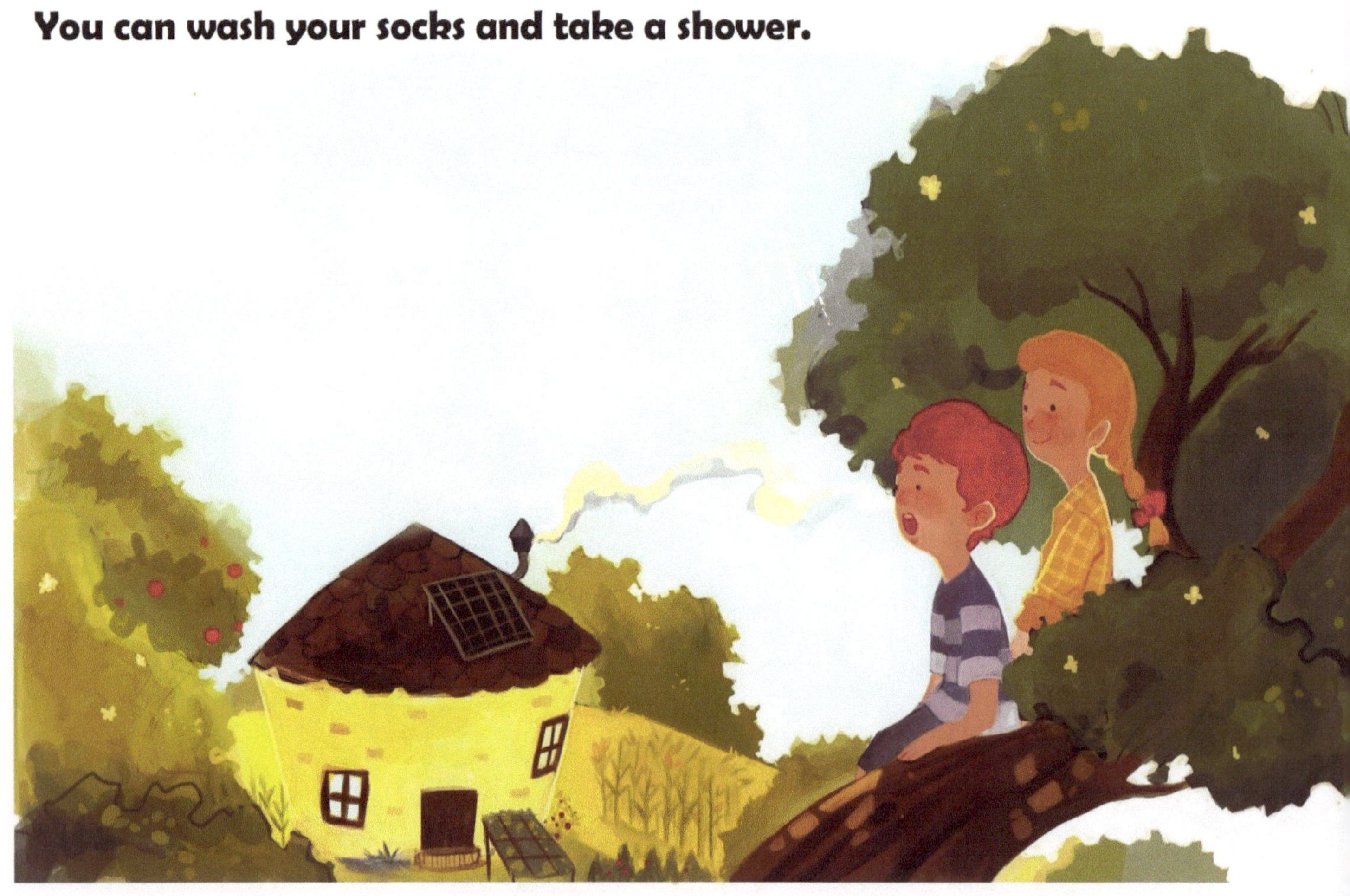

Watermelon! Watermelon! You make me go to the potty!
Except this one is different. It looks so dotty!
Is that a million biting ants?
Auntie please hurry! I don't want an accident in my pants.

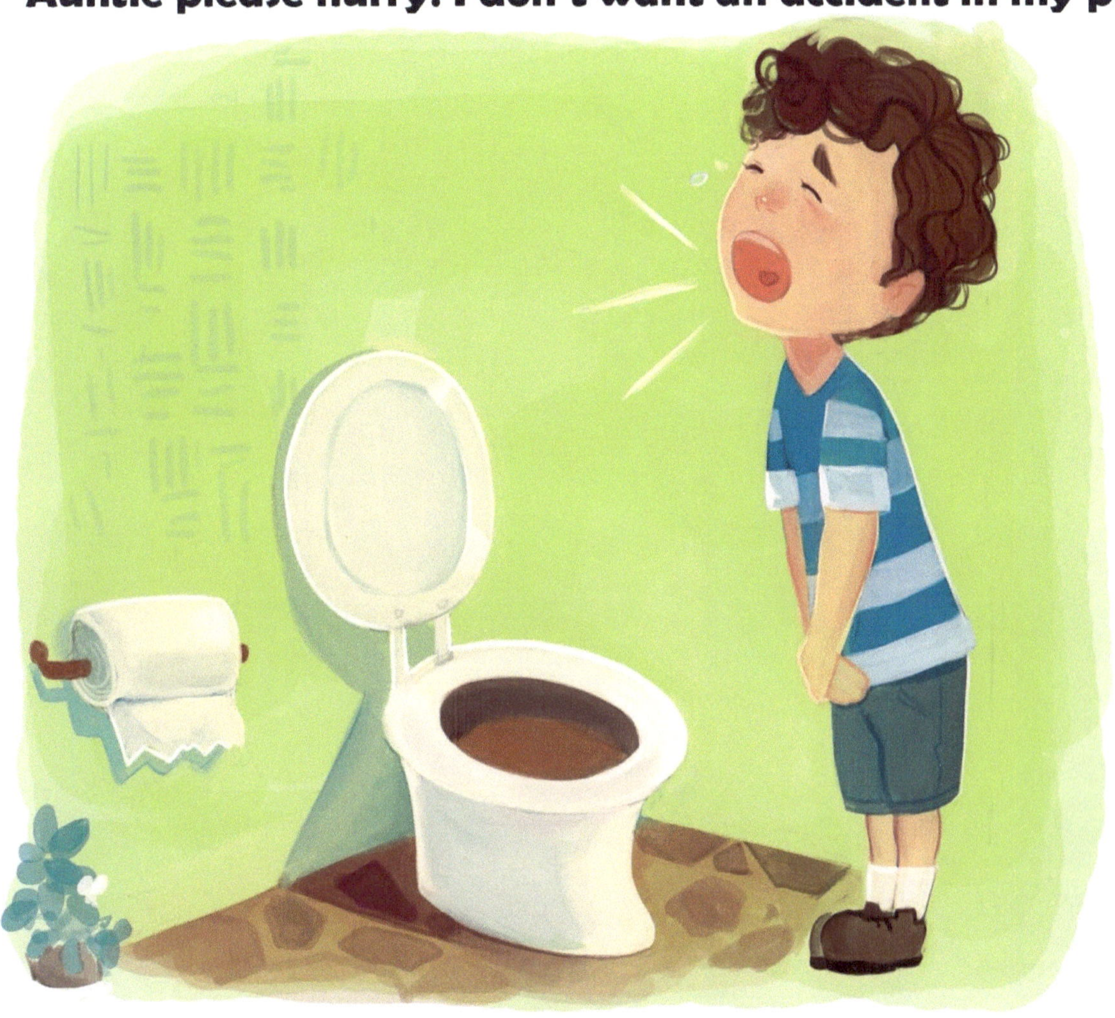

"Oh dear!
This is a composting toilet. No need to fear."
Slowly and cautiously, I move like a sloth down a tree.
By far the neatest toilet that I have ever gotten to see.

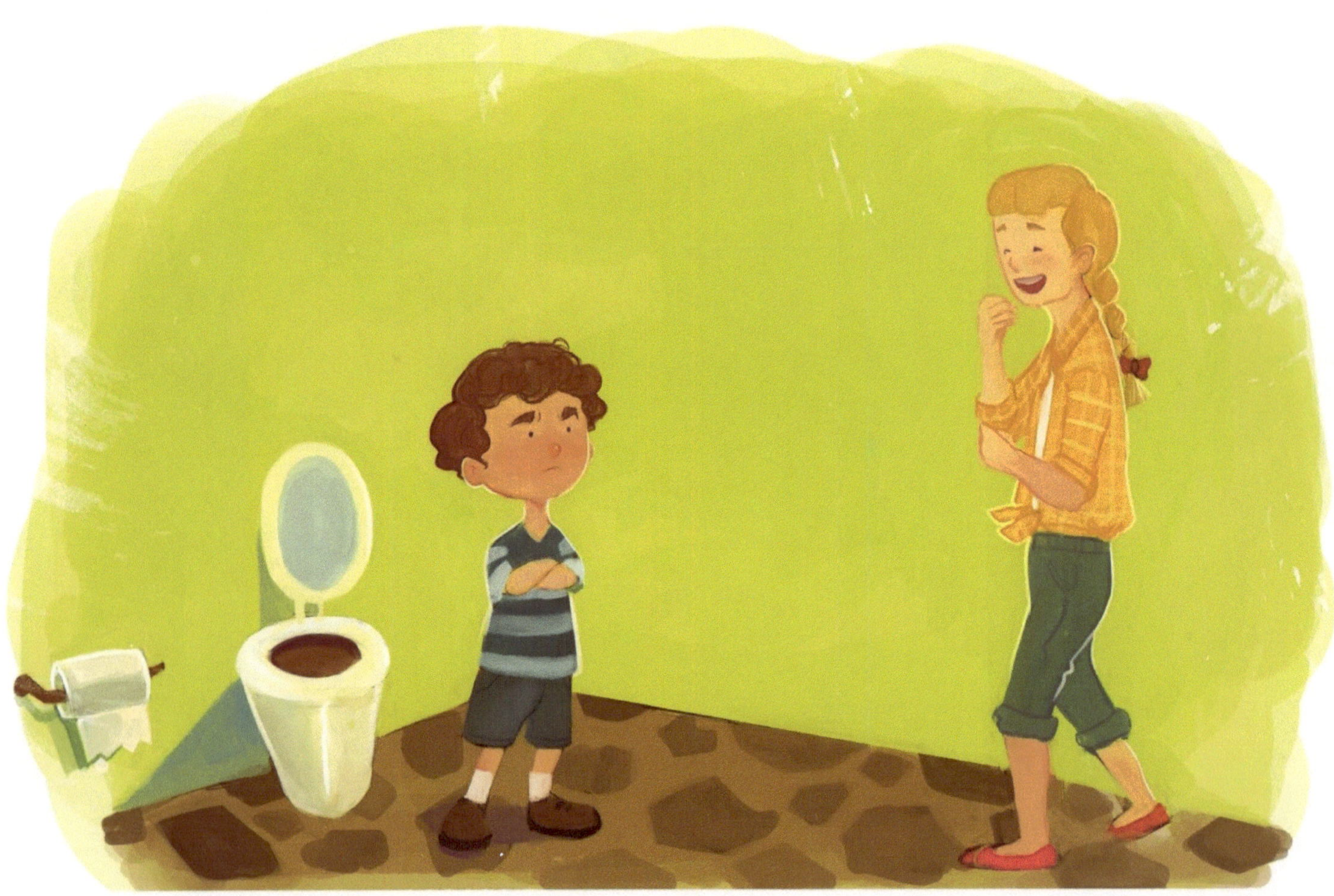

No water needed.
It's making food for the garden that is seeded.
No pollution as a result.
Let the whole Earth exult!

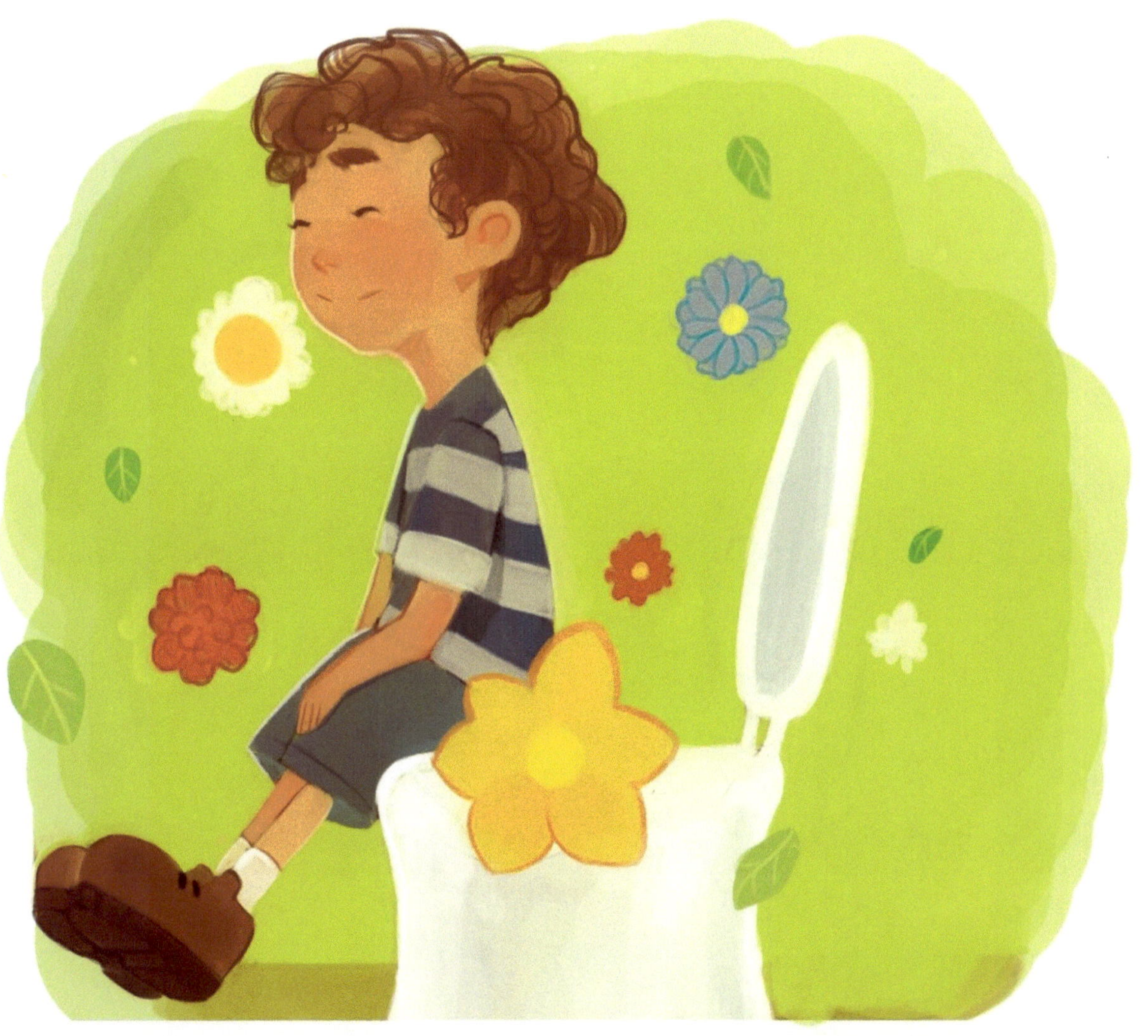

Dinner time! Dinner time! What yummy food shall we eat?
Auntie, can we have a hot dog, chicken nuggets, or some piece of meat?
"No, no dear. We choose to be kind to animals and eat only plants.
That way the animals can live happy lives and frolic and dance."

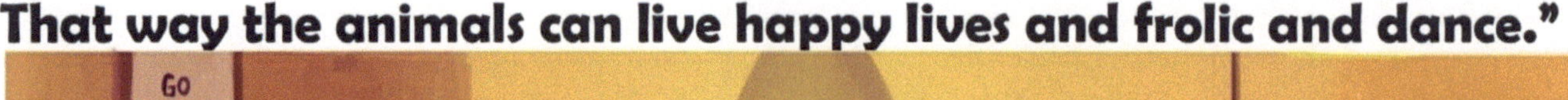

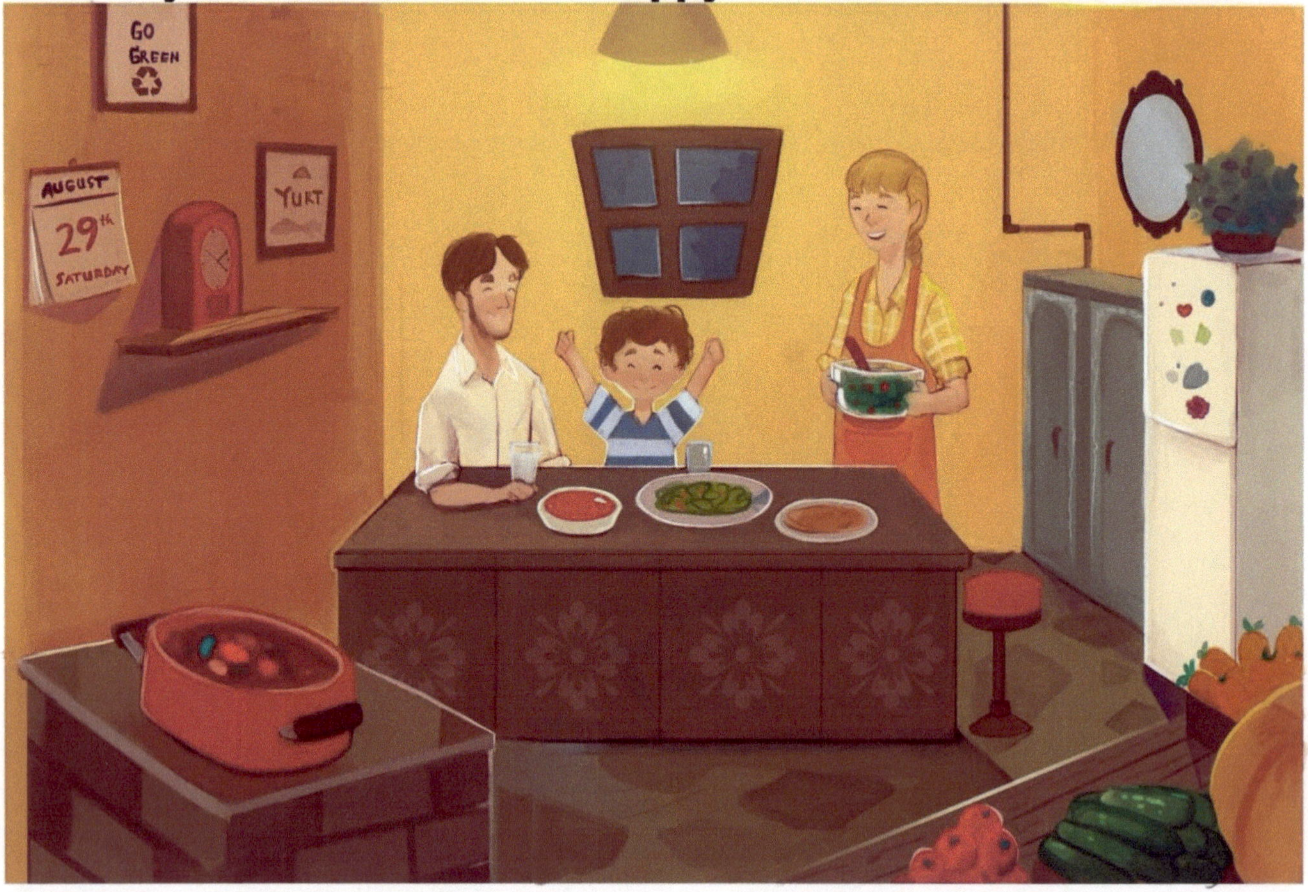

The sun shines on our bodies while we pick dinner from the plants.
It's like we are creating a joyful little dance.
The sun provides us with so much, who knew?
From helping plants grow, bringing joy, and drying the morning dew.

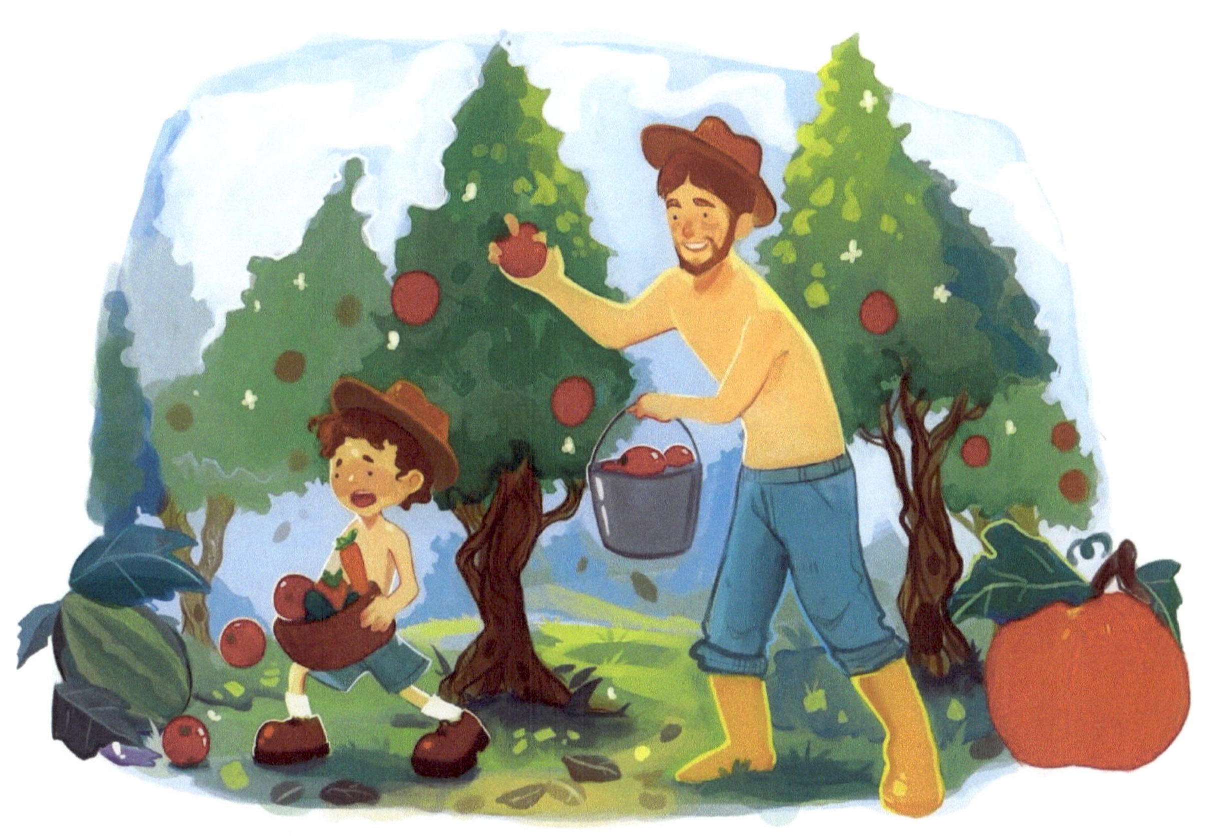

Broccoli, corn and potatoes.
Apples, cucumbers and tomatoes.

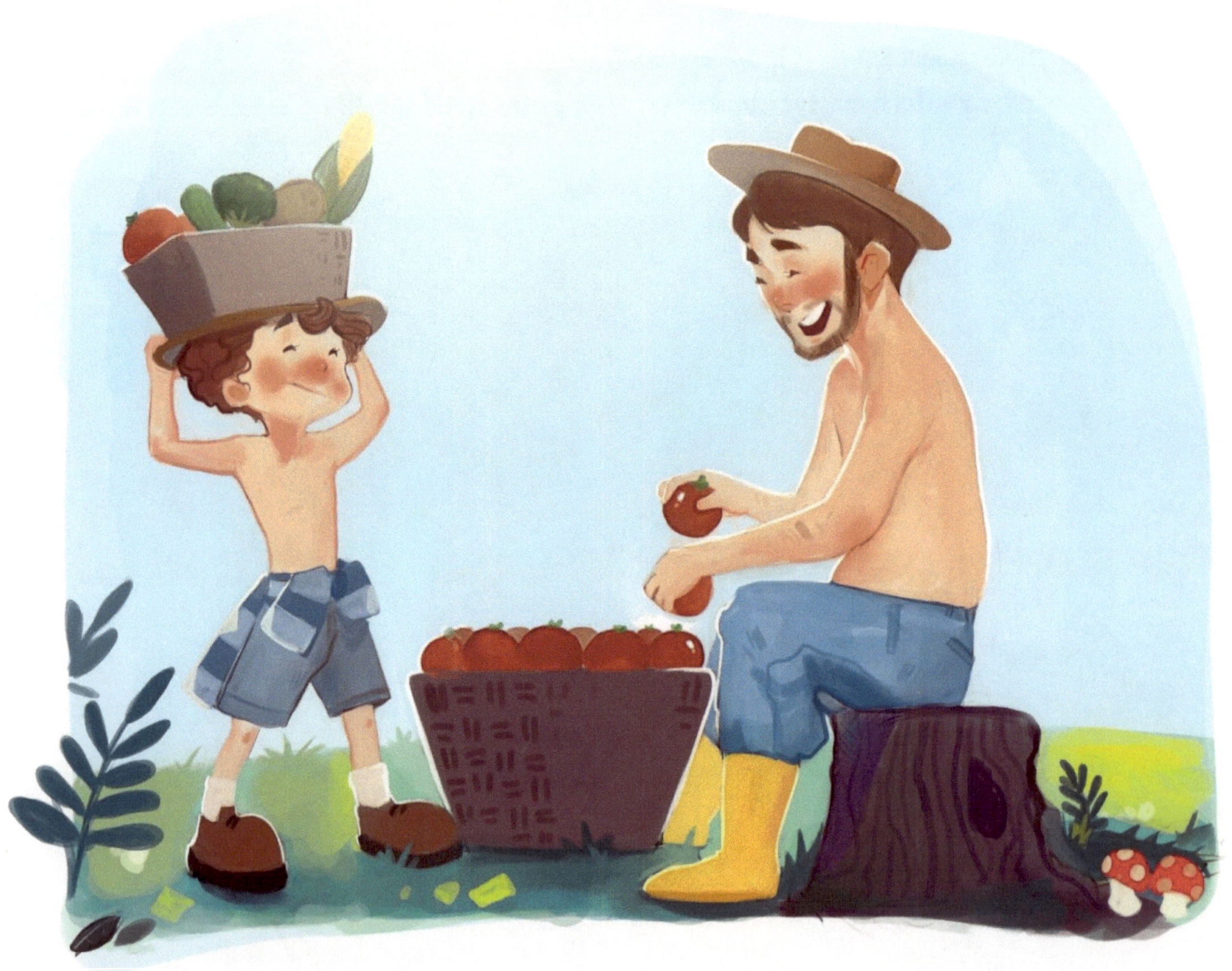

An herb spiral! An herb spiral! It's working in perfect harmony.
Bringing life to such great biodiversity.
Its shape is giving strength and power.
Plants are ready to take advantage of every sunshine and shower.

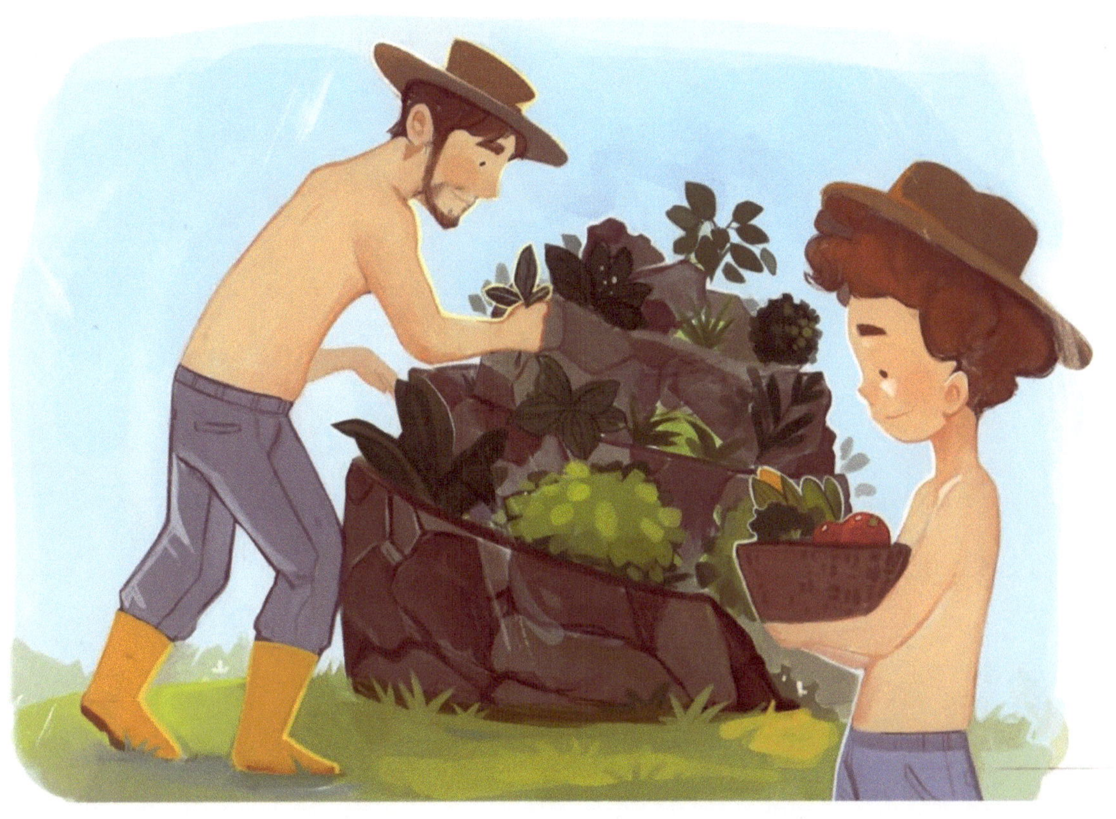

Auntie has prepared a delicious meal.
But first she says, "Let's take a moment to feel."
"Feel the love in your heart for the Earth and plants."
I close my eyes, but peak a glance.
I want to dive upon the food,
But mama always taught me not to be rude.

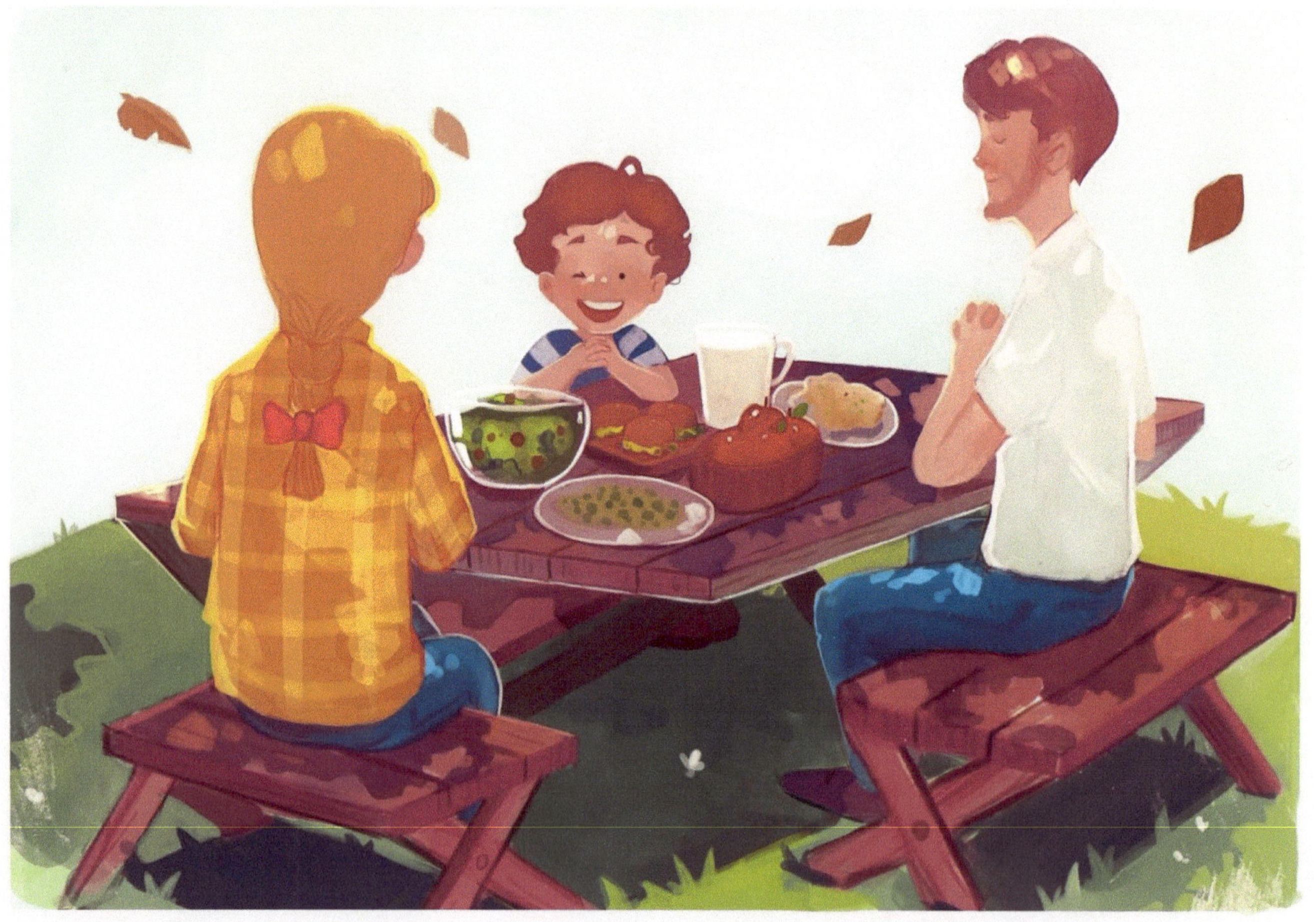

A hamburger that is tasty and yummy.
Auntie tells me it's a veggie patty; healthy for my tummy.
There's also milk made from almonds and not a cow.
Can you believe this? Wow!

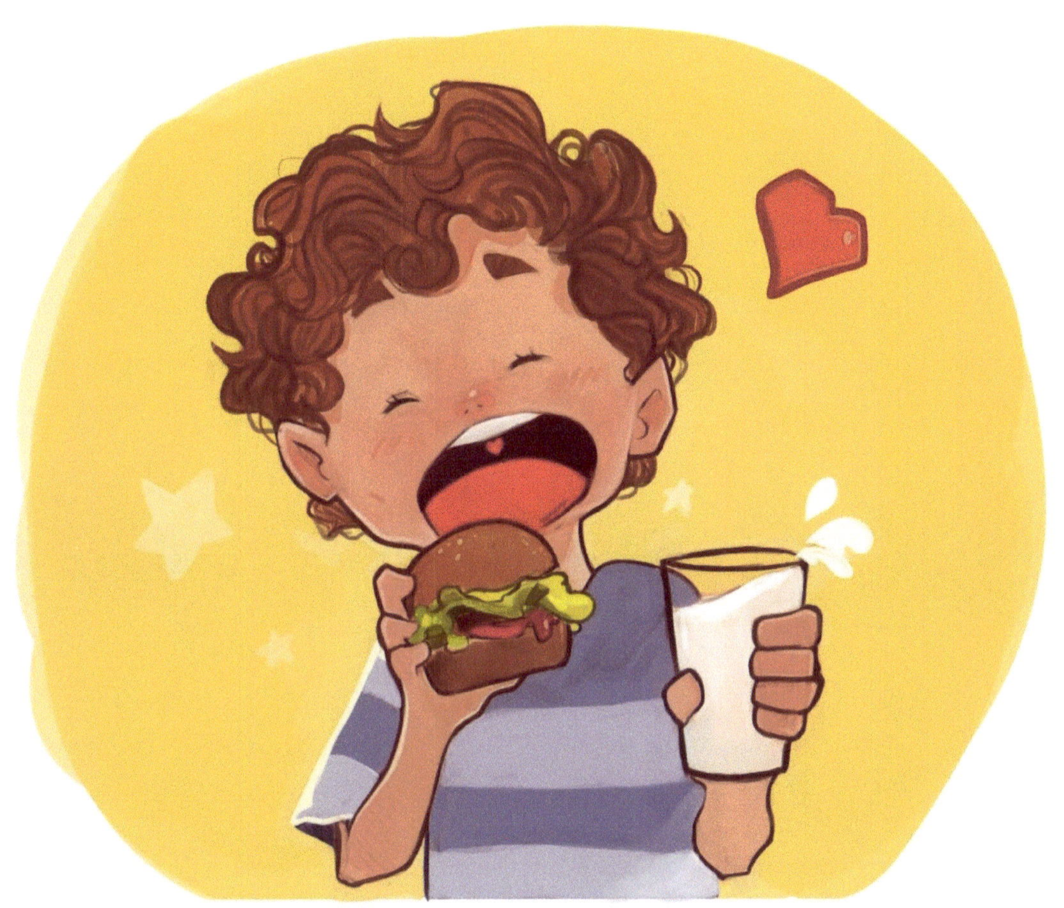

I bounce from each dish like a frog leaping from lily pad to lily pad.
I try potatoes a lot, veggie patty a bit, and almond milk a tad.
I never knew eating these different plants would be so rad.

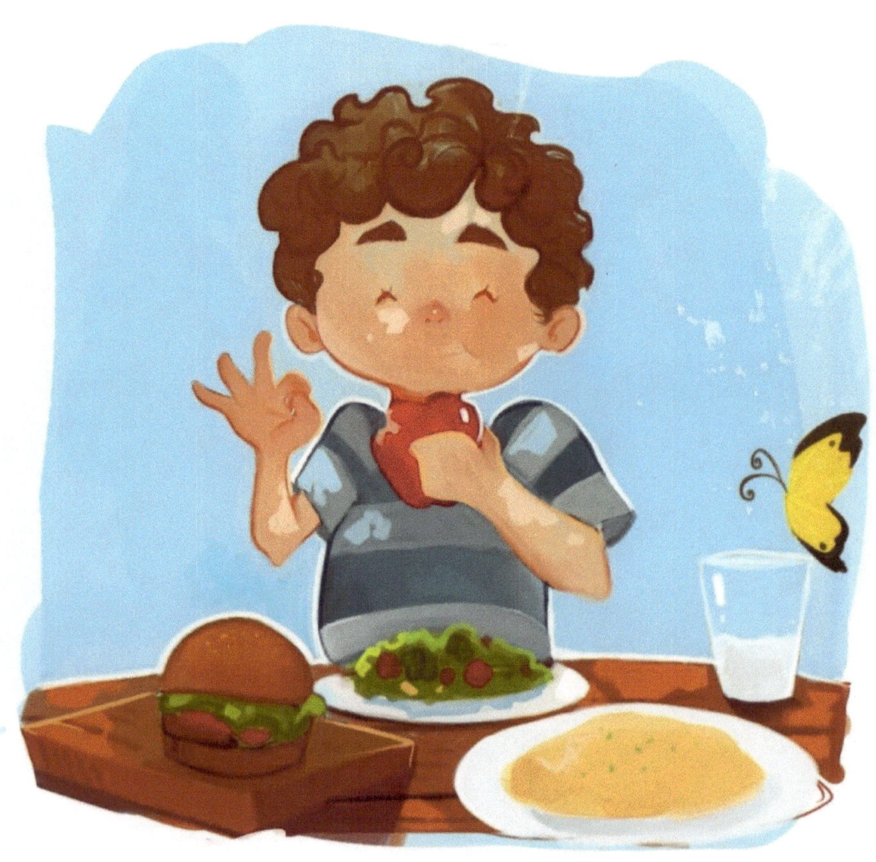

Oh, how I've eaten so many plants from the garden this meal.
I'm like a large hippopotamus, that's how I feel.
And, we didn't leave much on the table, except maybe a peel.

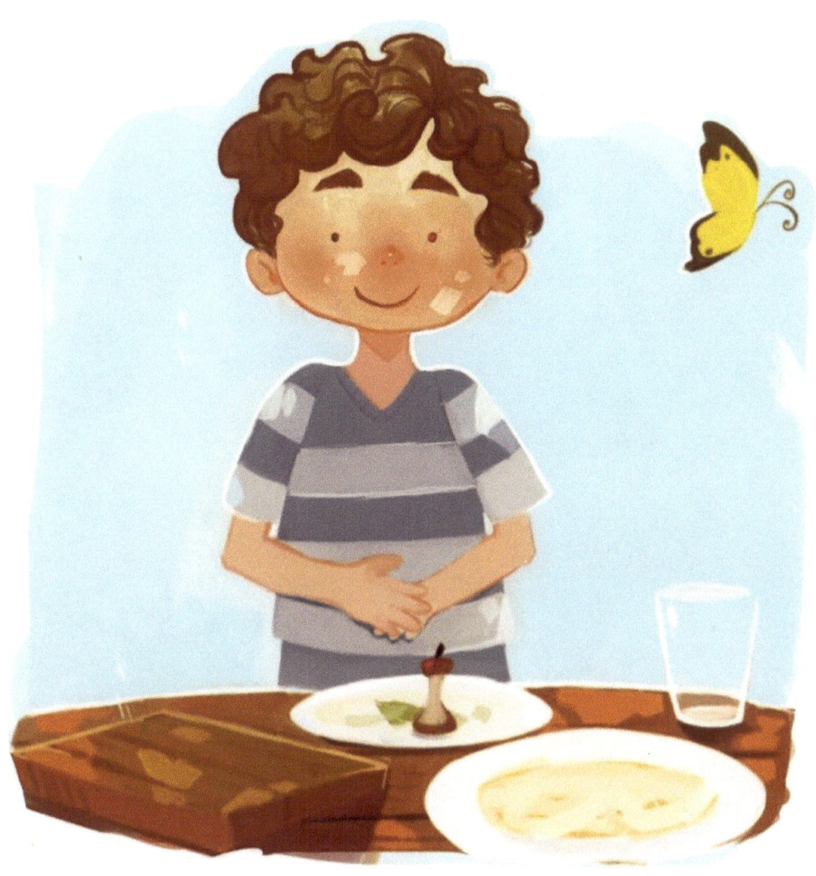

Bed time. Bed time. Time for some sleep.
Quiet time. Quiet time. No one say a peep.
I'm tucked in like a snail peeking out of my shell.
In the morning I may have a nice dream to tell.

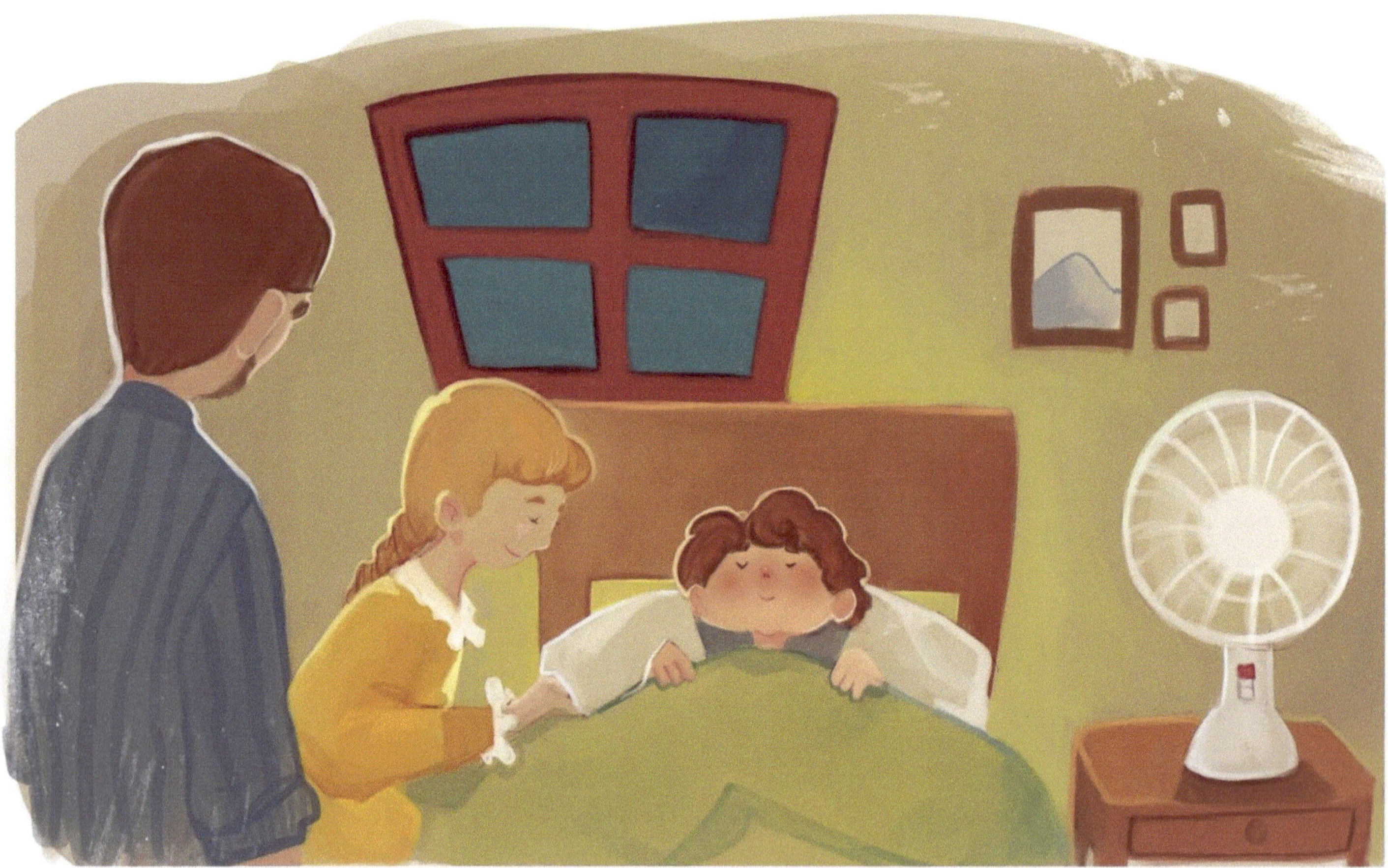

I awake to some noise outside in the yard.
I can almost hear some talking if I just listen hard.
I peek out the window and see the garden at night.
Suddenly I freeze like an opossum in the light.
The sunflower looks back at me from down on the right.
I must go and greet him out there tonight.

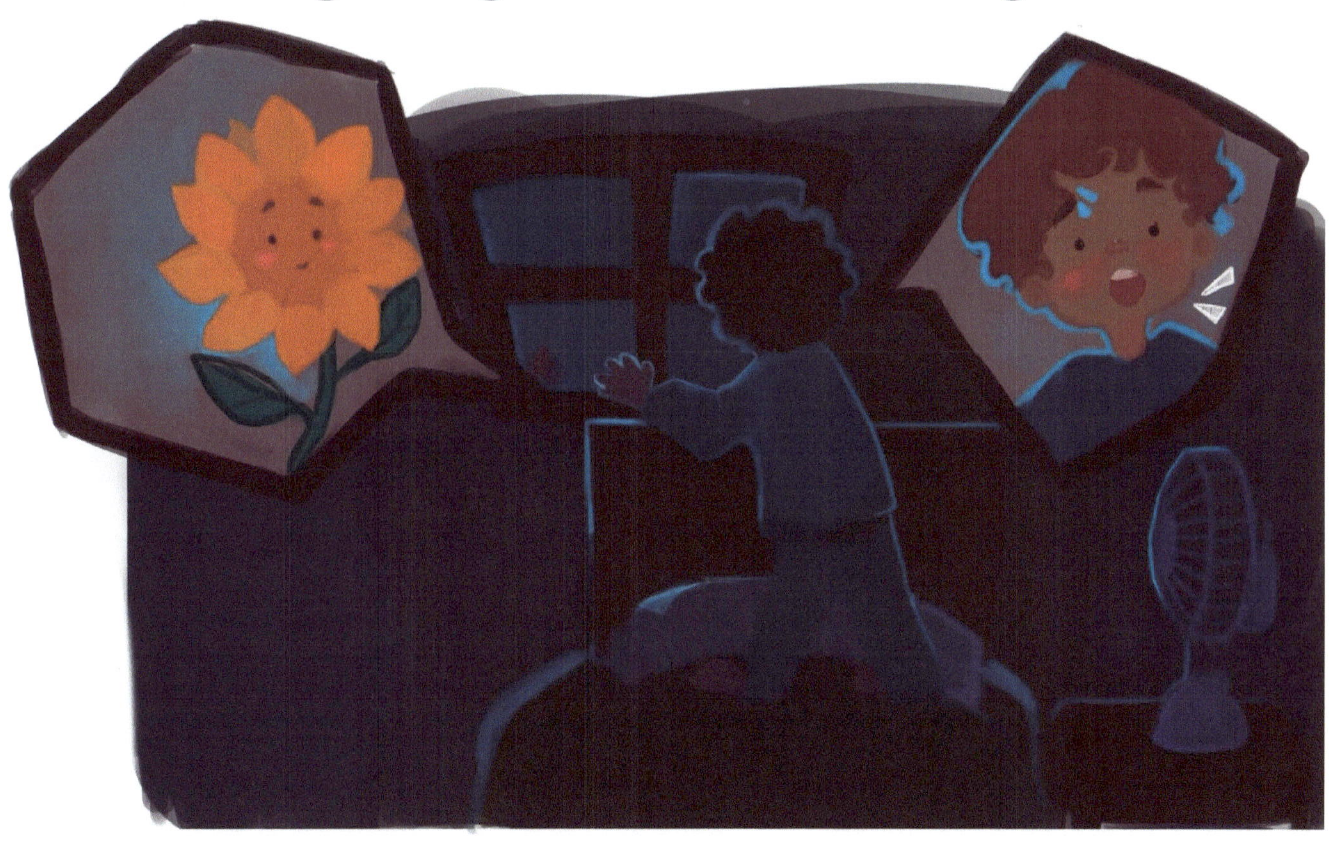

Sunflower and I meet.
Friends we quickly become with a gentle greet.
He teaches me to be kind to all on the Earth
The animals, plants, others and myself; so much we are worth.
Everything that is done has been done with compassion by Uncle and Auntie.
Looking around, it's in all that I see.

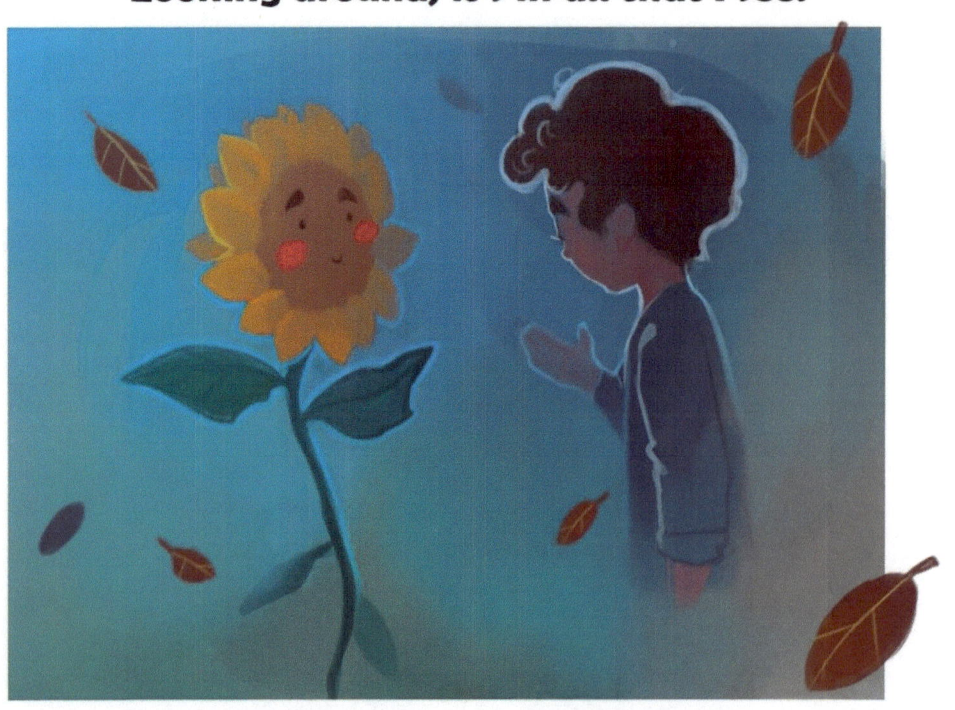

Sunflower teaches me that animals are not meant to be food.
They are our friends. Eating them would be rude.

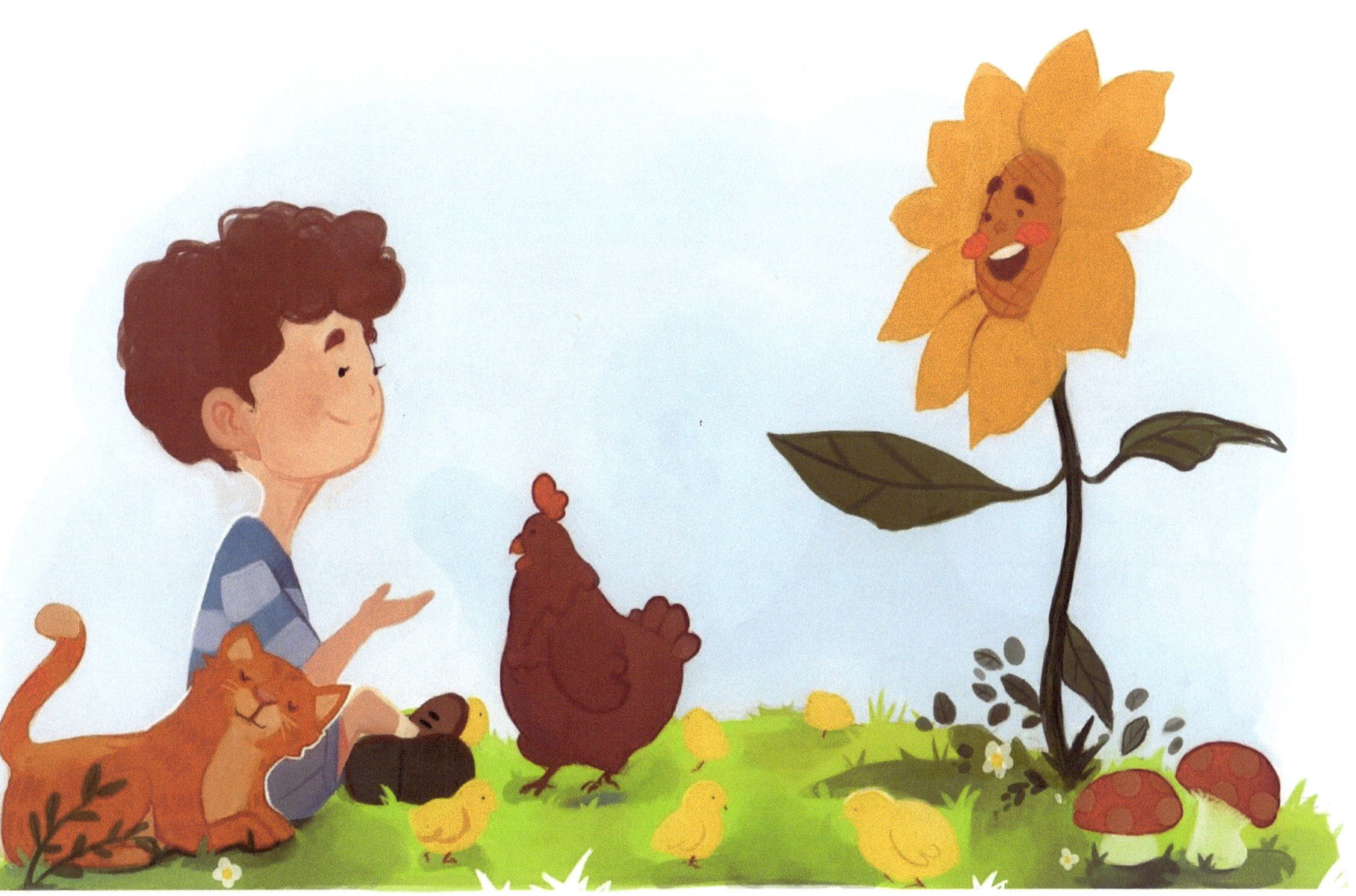

No hurt to the animals when we eat of the plants.
No hurt to myself. I'll just want to dance.
Sunflower tells me to be the best that I can be.
I can always do that when I choose to eat healthy.

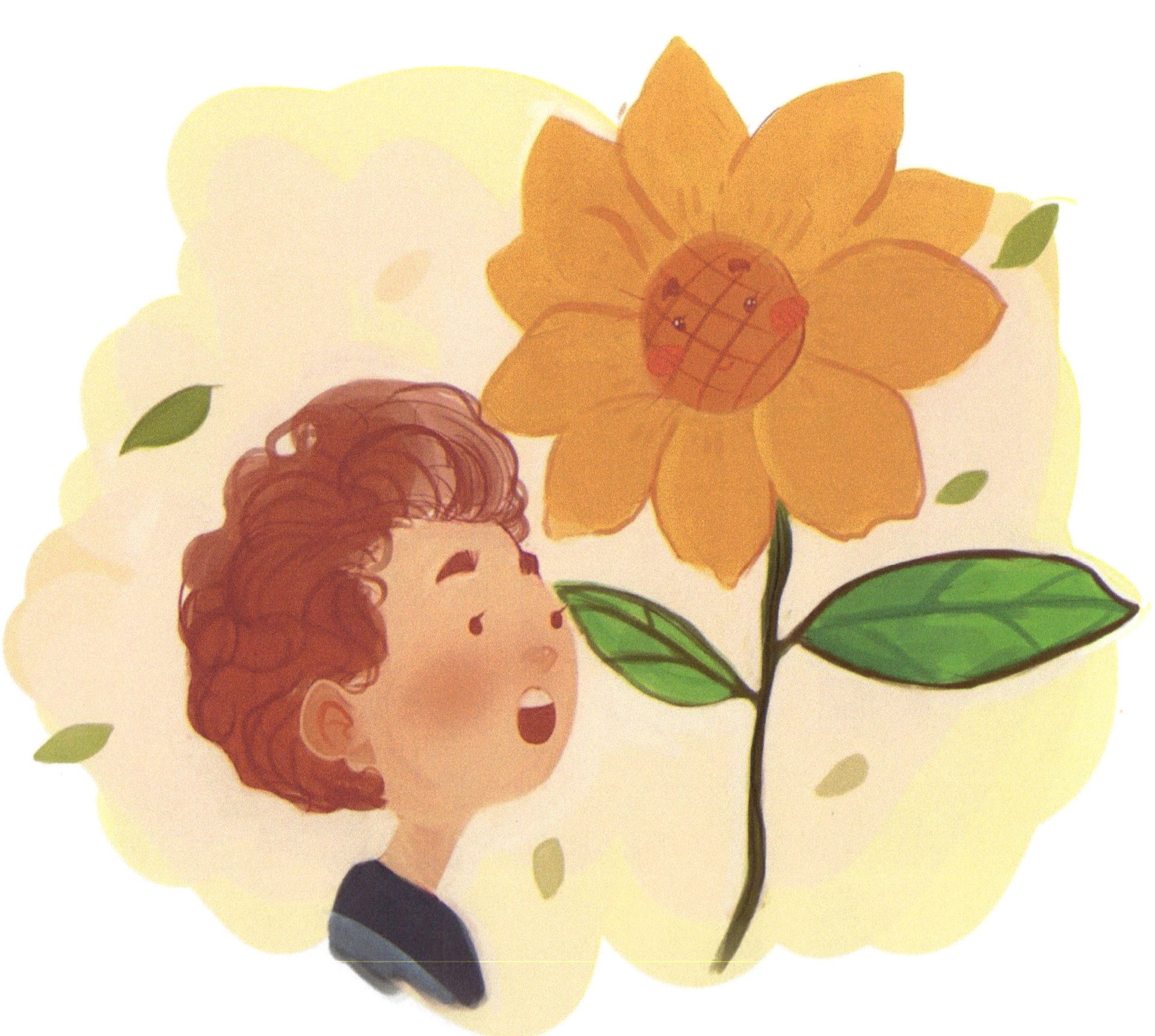

Ripe bananas: always enjoy.
And milks made of nuts or even soy.
A big 'ol salad topped with tomatoes.
And those oh so yummy sweet potatoes.

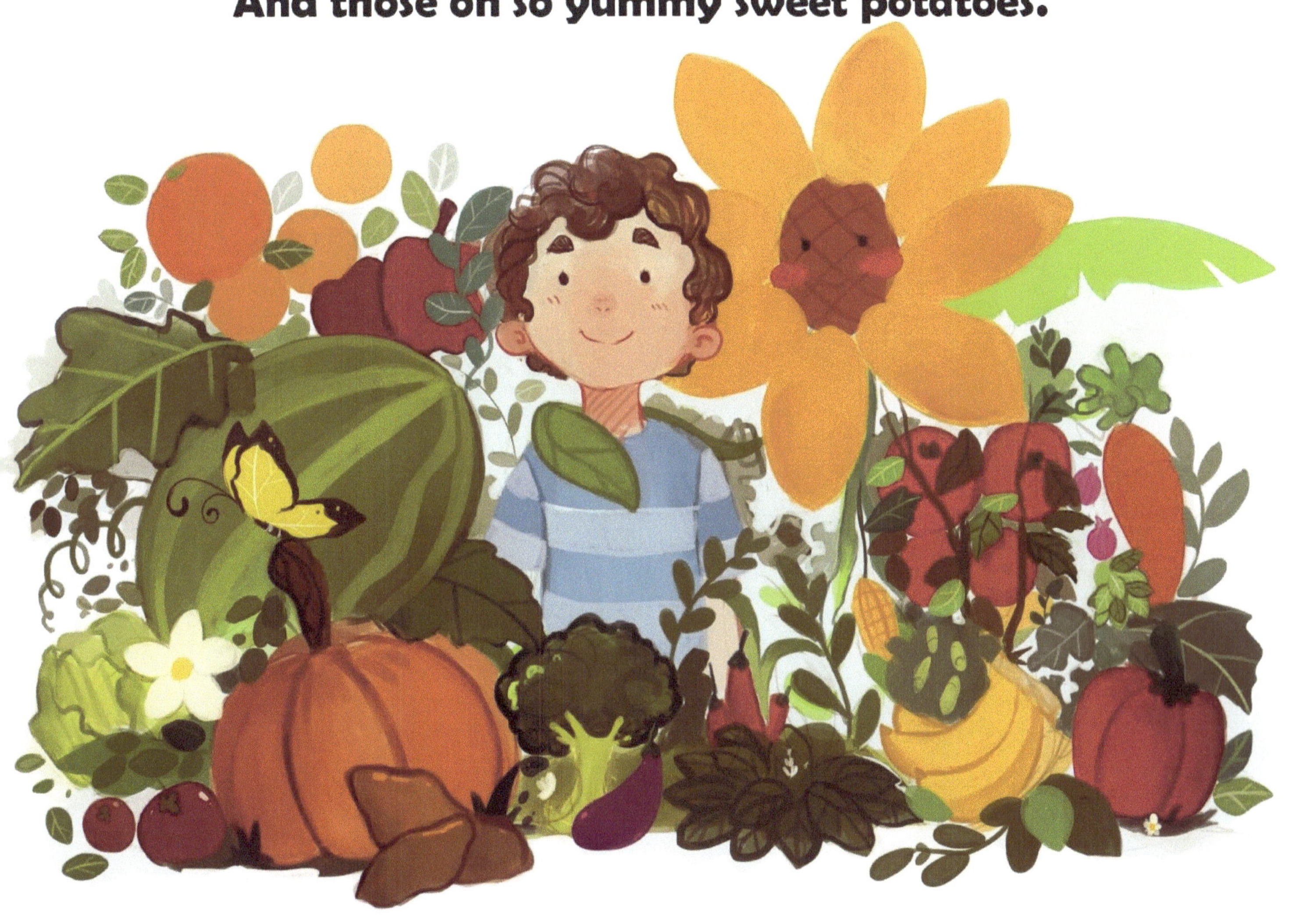

This information I shall always keep.
Now, I better get back to sleep.

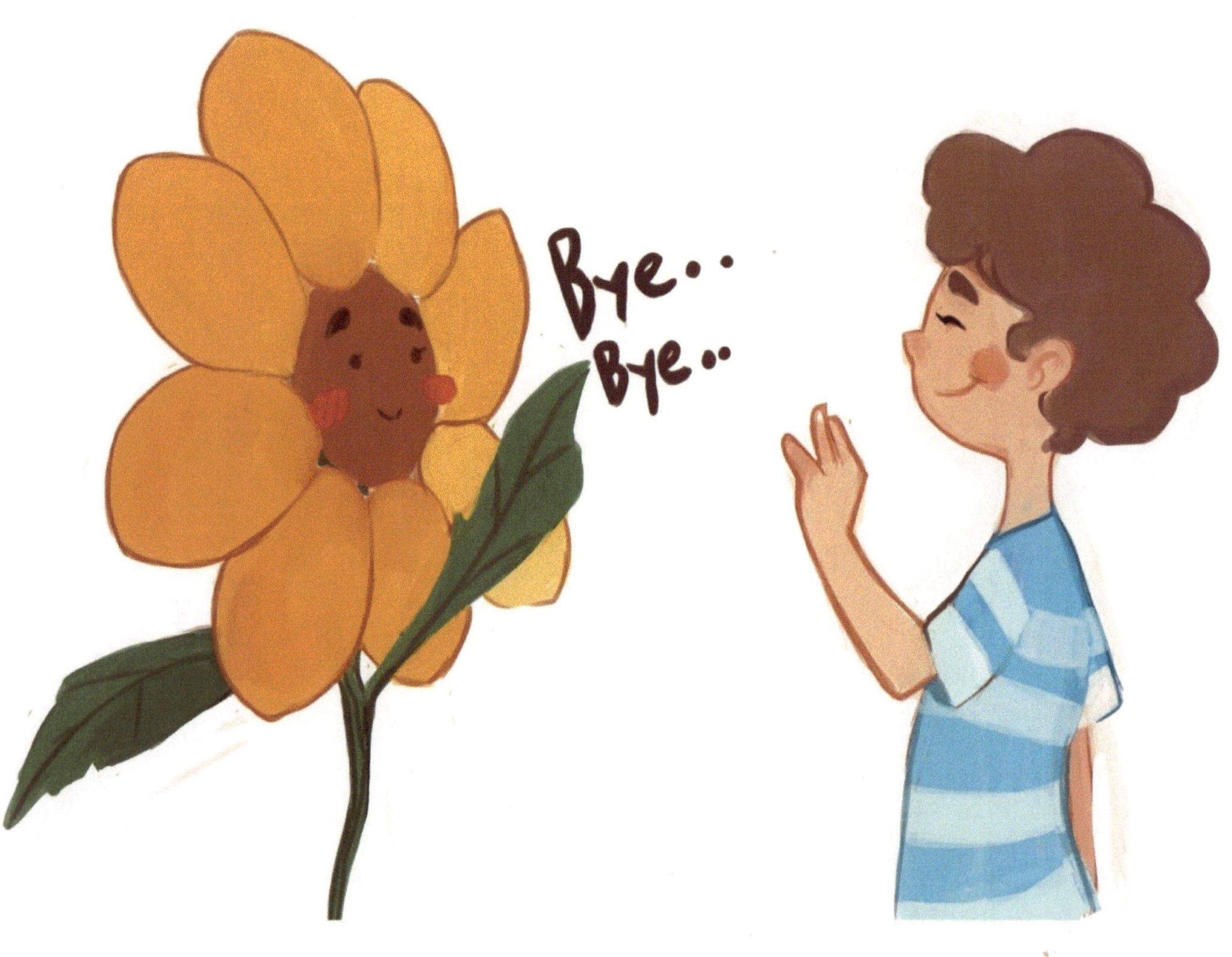

Like a fox stepping out of his den,
My eyes are blinking from the morning sun.
I reflect back upon my night and realize I have learned a ton.
Meeting Sunflower was super-duper fun!

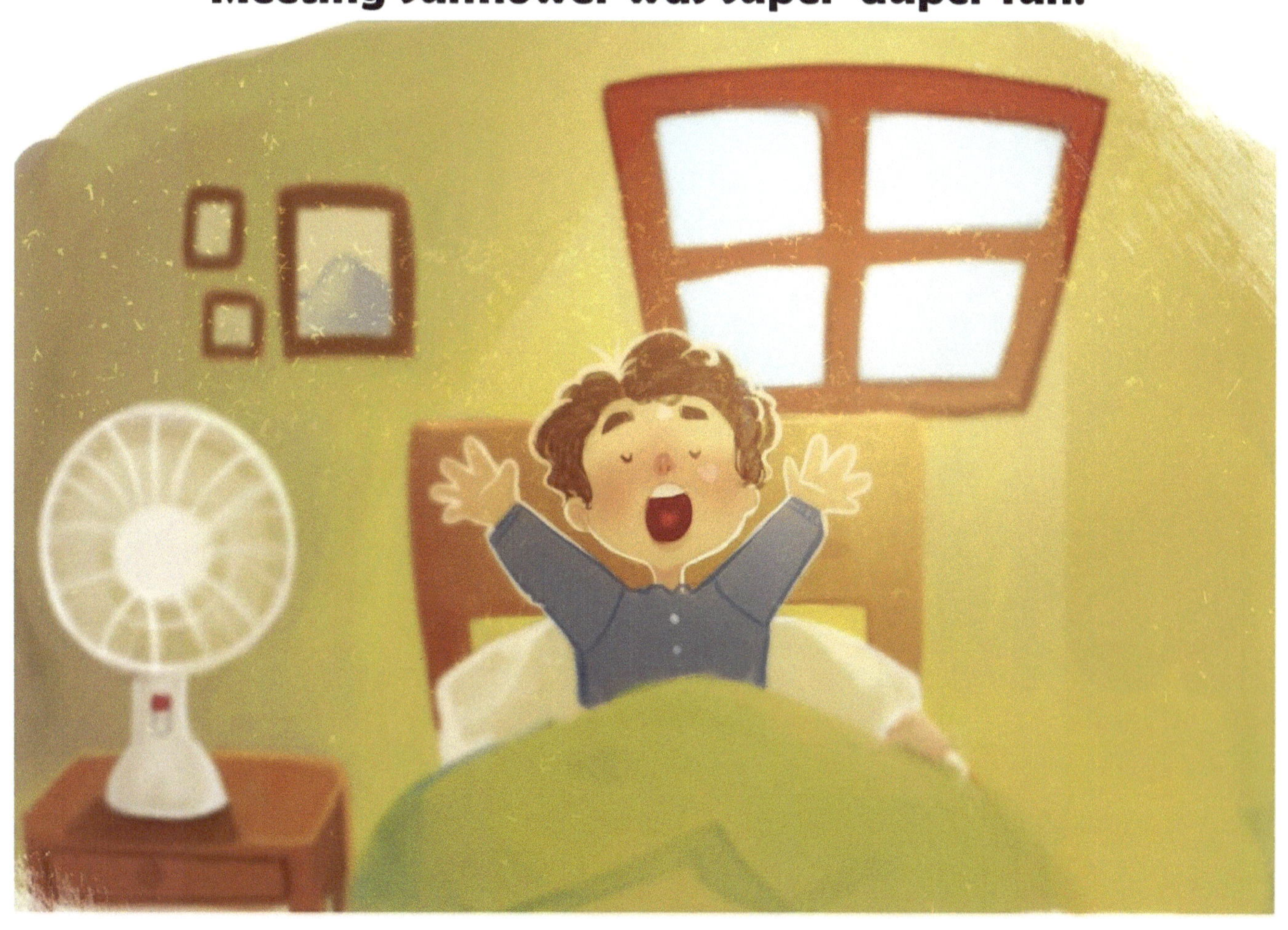

Stepping out of my room, what do I see?
Some weird acting by Uncle and Auntie.
"This is yoga," they share with me.
"Come and join us down on one knee.
We exercise our bodies and relax our minds.
Stretch like a cat, bend like a cobra, and reach high like the pines."

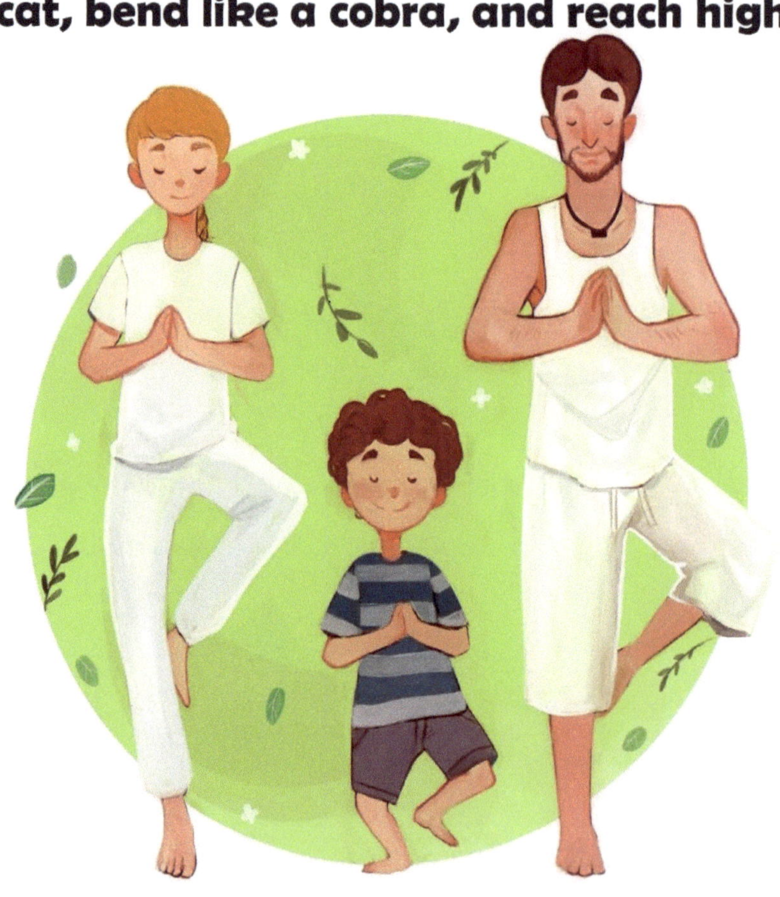

Just about time for mom to come get me.
But before that, Uncle says, "Come and see."
I'm given a baby sunflower to take home and plant.
Thank you! Thank you to the best uncle and aunt!

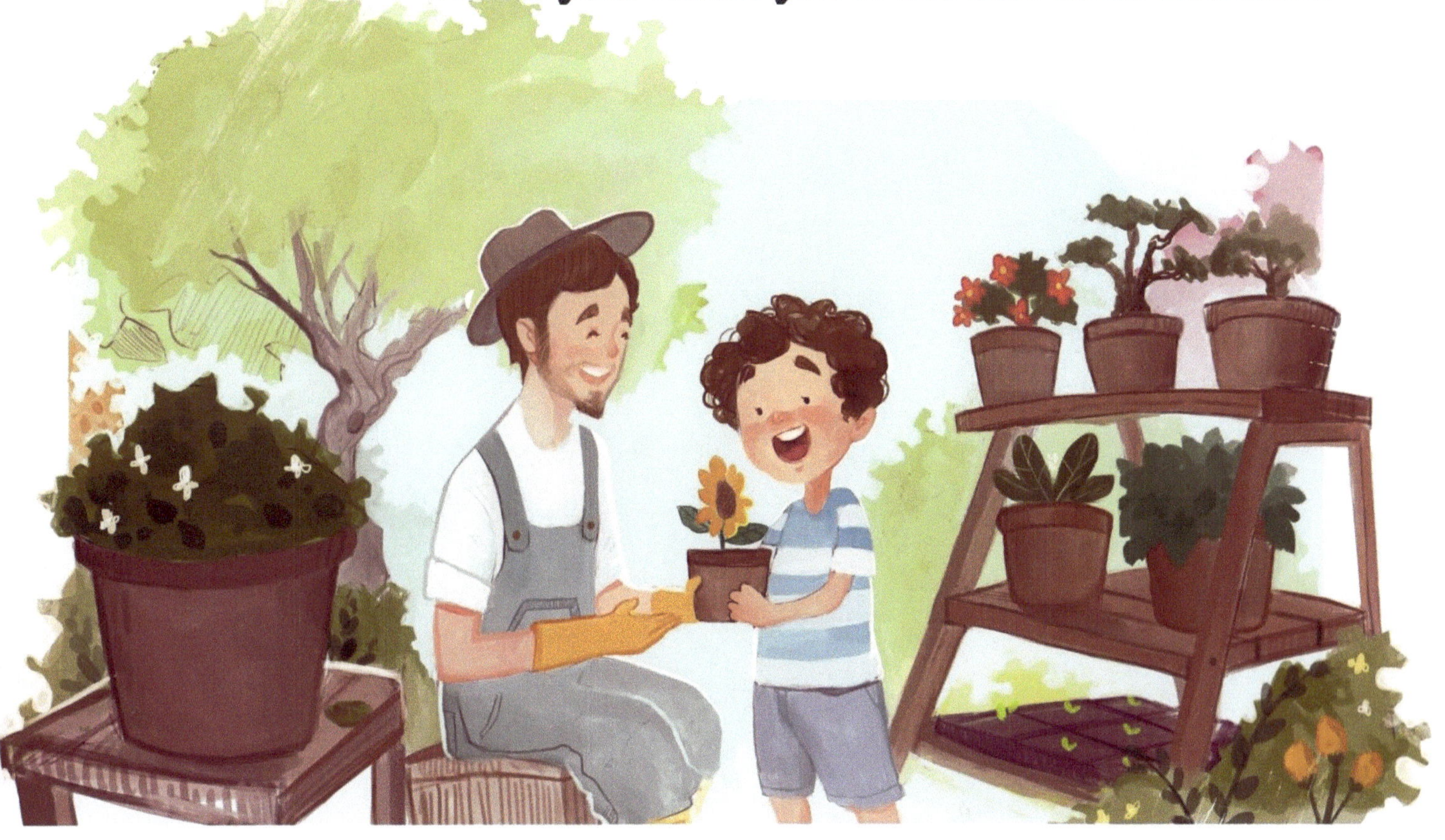

Driving home, mom asks what I would like to eat.
I tell her a big bowl of fruit would be a wonderful treat.
I'm holding baby sunflower tight in my hand.
I feel something tickle. It must be some sand.
I look down and wonder. What do I see?
Baby sunflower smiling back at me.

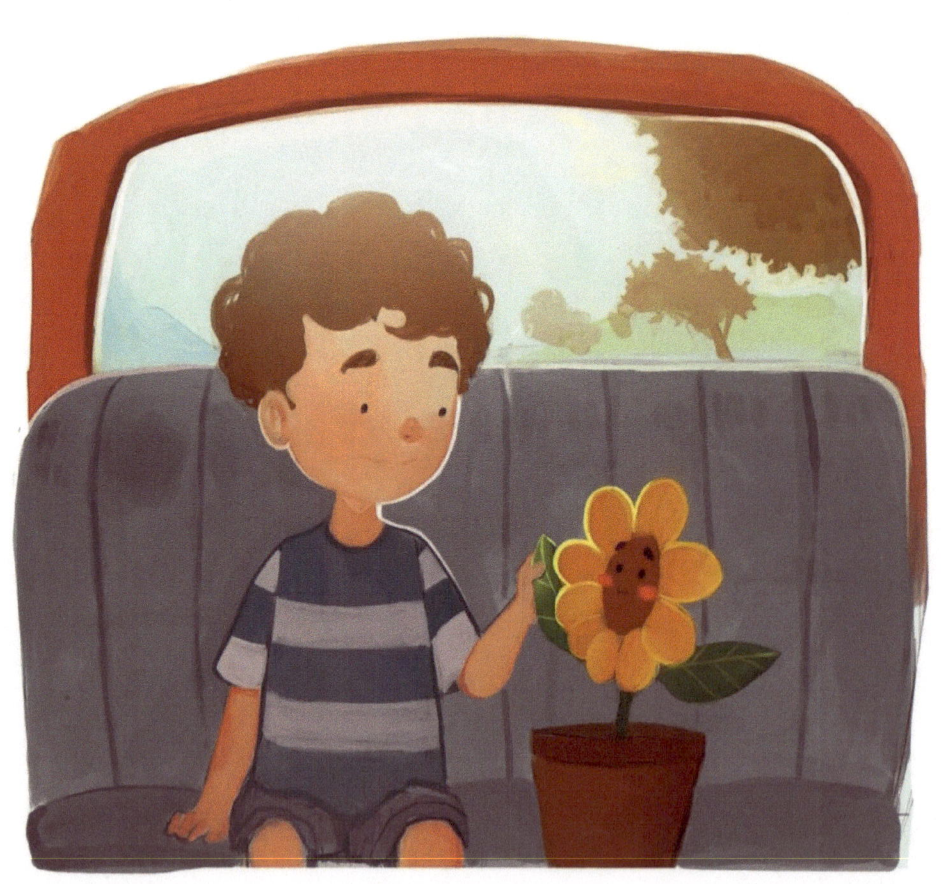

About the Author

Stephen Bedwell Jr. is a Certified Holistic Nutrition Practitioner who educates children to eat a healthy whole food plant-based diet and encourages children to be environmentally friendly. He achieves this through creative and poetic stories that tug at the hearts and minds of children. Stephen received a Master's Degree in Criminal Justice and has years of experience in child welfare where he has helped children and adults make positive life changes. In 2008, Stephen became interested in healthy living and quickly adopted a whole food plant-based diet and lifestyle. He does not shy away from carbohydrates and loves enjoying lots of fresh fruit.

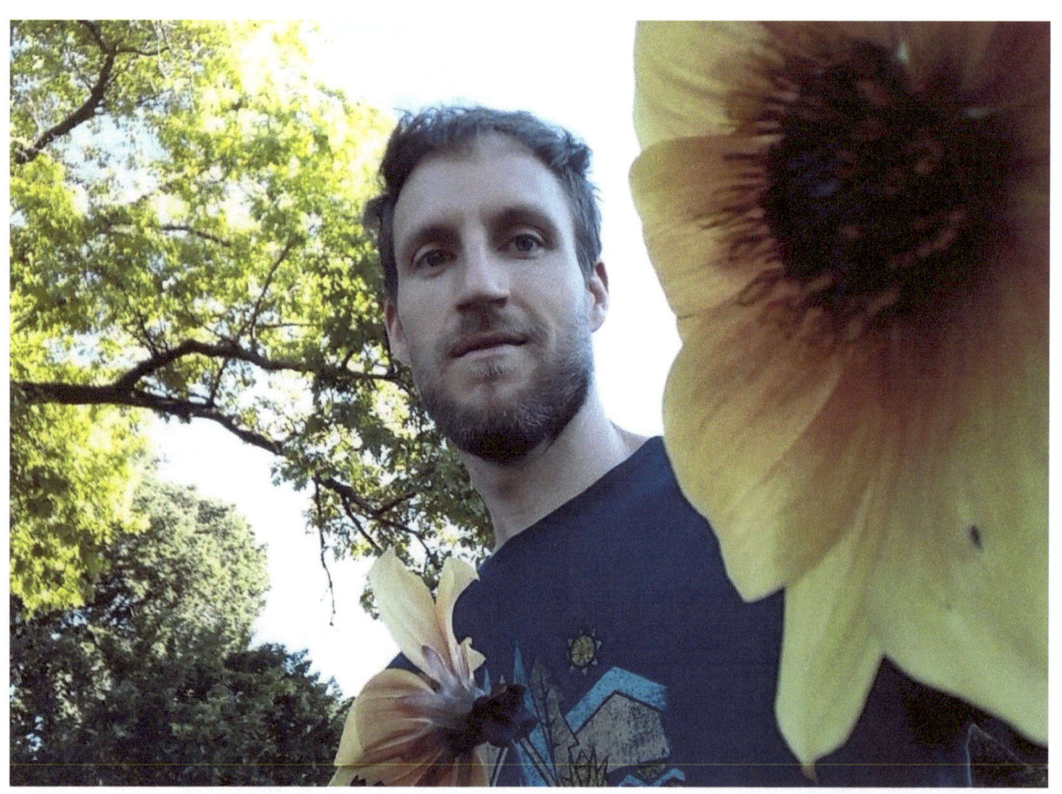

www.ingramcontent.com/pod-product-compliance
Lightning Source LLC
Chambersburg PA
CBHW040159240726
48664CB00002B/765